FAMILY
PLANNING

FAMILY PLANNING

Fundamentals for health professionals

Ann Cowper SRN, SCM, MTD, DN (London), ENB 900

Family Planning Nurse Specialist
Senior Midwifery Tutor
Worthing and Chichester School of Midwifery

Cyril Young MSc, FRCOG, MRCS, LCRP

Consultant Gynaecologist
Greenwich District Hospital, London

SECOND EDITION

SPRINGER-SCIENCE+BUSINESS MEDIA, B.V.

First published in 1981 by
Croom Helm Ltd

Typeset in 10/12 Palatino by
Photoprint, Torquay, Devon

ISBN 978-0-85664-907-3   ISBN 978-1-4899-3266-2 (eBook)
DOI 10.1007/978-1-4899-3266-2

British Library Cataloguing in Publication Data

Cowper, Ann, 1937–
    Family planning : fundamentals for health
    professionals.—2nd ed.
    1. Contraception 2. Family planning
    services
    I. Title II. Young, Cyril, 1942–
    613.9'4

Contents

Acknowledgements

Many people have contributed towards the successful completion of the first edition of this book, and we continue to be grateful for their support. The second edition has been hard on families especially at weekends and we thank them for their forbearance.

The text has been brought up to date and broadened to include the curriculum for the ENB 901 course for family planning nurses. In order to do this Norton Evans has kindly done additional illustrations. We have again used the condom cartoon 'Getting it on' by kind permission of Family Planning Sales Ltd.

The original team at the publishing HQ has taken a number of changes and moves. We wish them well in their new offices and would like to thank Christine Birdsall and all editorial and production staff involved with the book.

Preface

Our aim was quite clear when we agreed to write this book, and this was to cover in a single text, at the correct level, the syllabus for the Joint Board of Clinical Nursing Studies Course 900. The second edition has undertaken to produce further information to cover the present extended ENB 901 course.

Inevitably, having commenced on the task it quickly became obvious that this could develop into a life's work! The breadth and depth of the subject and its interrelating information are offered for the use of the family planning nurse and health professional, both trained and in training, with the hope that their basic needs will be met and their interest aroused for further reading.

The chapter on special needs fills, we trust, a neglected area in family planning training; and the problems which may be encountered with people from other countries is introductory information which is not easily available in this subject.

The use of the male prefix for doctors and female prefix for nurses and clients is to simplify the script and provide a smoother text for the reader. It does not imply that the authors believe that all family planning nurses and clients should be female and all doctors male; indeed we enjoy the fact that there is a considerable variety of both in this specialty.

Introduction

When Eve joined Adam, they started a series of population explosions that led to the rise and fall of many civilizations. Natural disasters, pestilence and war take their toll of the human race, as do changes in the economic climate, general living conditions and the health of the people. Contraception can play only a small part in modifying the birth rate, but it is an important part as it allows individuals the right to decide in advance on the size of their families more than it has ever been possible to do before.

Warnings of the need for population control have been sounded often enough in the past by eminent philosophers and scientists, and the practical pioneer work of the Family Planning Association has resulted in a keen awareness by HM Government of the need to provide scope for the practice of voluntary contraception. A great deal of ignorance still exists, and to cope with our changing society major efforts are being made by education, local and health authorities, with encouragement from the Department of Health and Social Security and the full support of the private and public sectors of the medical profession, to provide a wide range of facilities for sex education and advice on contraception.

There are now encouraging signs of a growing demand for these facilities and the future training of personnel for this specialized family planning service is of great importance. Working with people is normally colourful, and in the field of contraception it is as varied and interesting as could be wished. There are always new skills to be learnt and it is the aim of this book to ensure that any health professional involved in this field is aware of the full range of responsibilities entailed and has the relevant theoretical and practical information to do the job with confidence and pleasure.

1

The needs of the individual for contraception

The fundamental urge to procreate is dynamic, making itself felt long before the mantle of maturity descends upon us. The arguments which arise when sex education is mentioned are as old as history itself, but the more progressive the country becomes the greater the need for its citizens to be well informed on matters relating to the responsible attitudes on sex.

1.1 FACILITIES FOR EDUCATION

Apart from the natural environment of the home into which the child is born and from which it absorbs its first impressions of life, self-knowledge is attained in a number of different ways.

The family

Small children comparing their genitalia with their brothers, sisters and friends indicate the first signs of sexual awareness with which most parents are familiar. In well adjusted families this natural curiosity is sensitively responded to with brief spells of intelligent support at the same level of the child's playful observations. In fact, it is interesting to note that the human species starts early to prepare itself for reproduction. Early development of the embryo shows a strange awareness of the need for perpetuity by developing its gonads before all the other major organs to make sure of the reproduction of the species! Small wonder then that young people begin to experiment with the life force within them at puberty before they are fully conscious of the value of good relationships and the responsibility of parenthood.

Schools

Attempts by Education Authorities, supported by medical experts, to provide a well balanced sex education in schools have not, for various reasons, met with the success they deserve. The growing awareness of the need for contraception by adult couples is encouraging and the demand for advice by the young at doctors' surgeries and family planning clinics offers an opportunity to widen the scope of sex education and teach some essential body mechanics. Formal education in schools needs to be reconsidered, as a great deal of ignorance still exists and children should be made aware that they can receive individual help in any family planning clinic. If the subject of contraception is separated from other school subjects and dealt with by an outsider, it is much more difficult to engage the interest of the children and offer them meaningful information. The subject should, where possible, be included in discussion with teachers who are well known and respected by the children.

General practitioners

Doctors in general practice can be the source of help and advice on contraception to anyone who seeks their help. Their awareness of the needs of the young makes them sensitive to an oblique approach for information. They will be able to assess the needs of the girl at whatever age, within her family setting. It will be necessary for them to reassure the younger girl who may be concerned about the family's reactions that confidentiality will be observed.

Many general practitioners have now extended their services by employing a family planning nurse to help them in the practice. This should ensure that a full service is provided in which all methods including the more frequently used non-medical techniques can be discussed and understood without embarrassment. Nurses may also provide counselling and support following termination.

Publicity and the media

The media are very conscious of their responsibility to the public to follow advances and controversies in different fields of medical research, and contraception is a particularly vital area of interest. A healthy watch-dog attitude seems to have developed and, whilst new methods of contraception are eagerly discussed, some failures are criticized with undue emphasis and severity in the absence of all the facts. This sometimes leads to unnecessary anxiety which is quickly reflected in the clinic attendances. The media certainly serves as a useful source of publicity, and the general public is kept well informed of developments and the kind of care it should expect to receive from clinics and surgeries.

The antenatal mother

During her first pregnancy a woman receives intensive health education of various kinds. It may the the first time she has experienced a full medical examination. Several tests are performed such as blood tests and scanning, and a cervical smear is usually taken at the first visit. Subsequently, the mother will become aware of a wide range of facilities for health care which are available to her. In addition she has the opportunity to discuss contraception and the advantages to be gained by spacing her future family.

1.2 FACILITIES FOR RECEIVING CONTRACEPTIVE ADVICE

Facilities for receiving advice and contraception are available without charge through many channels, but are still only used by a small number of the sexually active population. Perhaps this is due to the negative necessity for using contraception with which individuals find they are confronted. If freedom from unwanted pregnancy could be achieved by non-intervention the remainder of this text would become unnecessary. It is difficult to convince some people that controlling family size is an advantage when they receive child allowances, housing improvements and the pleasure of having a large loving family in their old age.

Local authority clinics

Family planning clinics are situated in all the health districts, some in community health centres and some in hospitals. The clinics give free advice and free contraception on demand. Working in the clinics are receptionists, clerical staff, doctors who hold family planning certificates awarded by the Joint Committee on Contraception

(or have the Family Planning Association certificate which pre-
ceded it), and Registered General Nurses who hold the English
National Board certificate 901 (previously 900 or Family Planning
Association certificate). In clinics where training in family planning
is carried out, trainee doctors and nurses may also be involved in
seeing those coming for advice. All trainees are closely supervised
and instructed but no one attending the clinic is obliged to have a
trainee in attendance.

Clinics in hospitals

Most district general hospitals have a family planning clinic on a
full or part-time basis. In most cases hospital patients can get
information, on request, about their local family planning clinic,
where staff may be better able to give specific sexual advice relating
to post-operative or medical conditions.

General practitioners

Many doctors in general practice give excellent contraceptive
advice to their patients. A few GPs have no background training in
family planning and prefer to send the patient to a local clinic.
Those responsible for the training of medical students are now
more aware of the need to prepare them for this role, but it is still a
very small part of their training in obstetrics and gynaecology. The
DRCOG examination is attempting to remedy this position, but as
this postgraduate training is unfortunately not essential for a GP
appointment there are still some who are unable to provide a
satisfactory contraceptive service.

Whilst GPs were initially unhappy about undertaking the extra
responsibility of sexual advice and contraception, it has now
become accepted by them as part of their role and they are well
remunerated by their family practitioner committees.

Domiciliary service

This service still exists in some districts where the population need
is high. Unfortunately the high cost of providing domiciliary care
makes it vulnerable to economic attack. People are referred to
domiciliary services by social workers, health visitors, hospitals,
private termination agencies and general practitioners.

The domiciliary staff is usually small, consisting of a doctor and nurse team, with administrative and clerical staff where possible to provide back-up support. The sort of people who benefit from this personal service are mothers with large families, the handicapped client, some non-English speaking immigrants and those who require constant encouragement as they are not well motivated to attend the family planning clinic on a regular basis.

The success of the domiciliary team is difficult to measure, they sometimes have to make enormous efforts to maintain good individual contraception: it is a hard job but frustration is mixed with some colourful and rewarding experiences.

Well women clinics

With the expansion of the well women service in preventive medicine a wider age group is seeking regular health checks.

During the intimate conversations associated with these visits and examinations information may be sought on contraception and accurate advice should be readily available. Contraceptive and sexual practices alter with increasing age and these may require full discussion with an informed health professional.

Private

Some people seek private contraceptive advice and there are many excellent doctors who practise both privately and in the NHS. The continuity of care under the one adviser has advantages.

2

Female body mechanics

It is the aim of this section that only the appropriate essentials of reproductive anatomy and physiology should be included so that the normal is well understood and common deviations recognized. The implication of this knowledge to the giving of contraceptive advice is included. In addition the ageing processes related to reproduction are mentioned to assist those providing well women services.

The more elaborate material, omitted here, may be found in textbooks written for that purpose listed in the bibliography.

2.1 THE VULVA

The general appearance of the external female genitalia is shown in Figure 2.1. Note that the main skin folds of the labia majora have smaller labia minora within. The latter join in a small hood or prepuce which covers the clitoris. During vaginal examination it is important that this very sensitive area is avoided to prevent discomfort. The labia join at the fourchette to form the anterior boundary of the perineum (the area which separates the vaginal introitus from the anus, consisting of strong muscle tissue which helps to maintain the position of the intra-abdominal contents). The perineum may be scarred as the result of a tear or episiotomy associated with previous childbirth. Occasionally there may be a definite deficiency, incomplete healing or tender puckering which may have been caused by less than perfect surgical reconstruction. In rare instances scarring may be found around the clitoris as a result of the ritual circumcision practised by some cultures. (The operation is thought to increase fidelity and reduce the level of female sensation and arousal.)

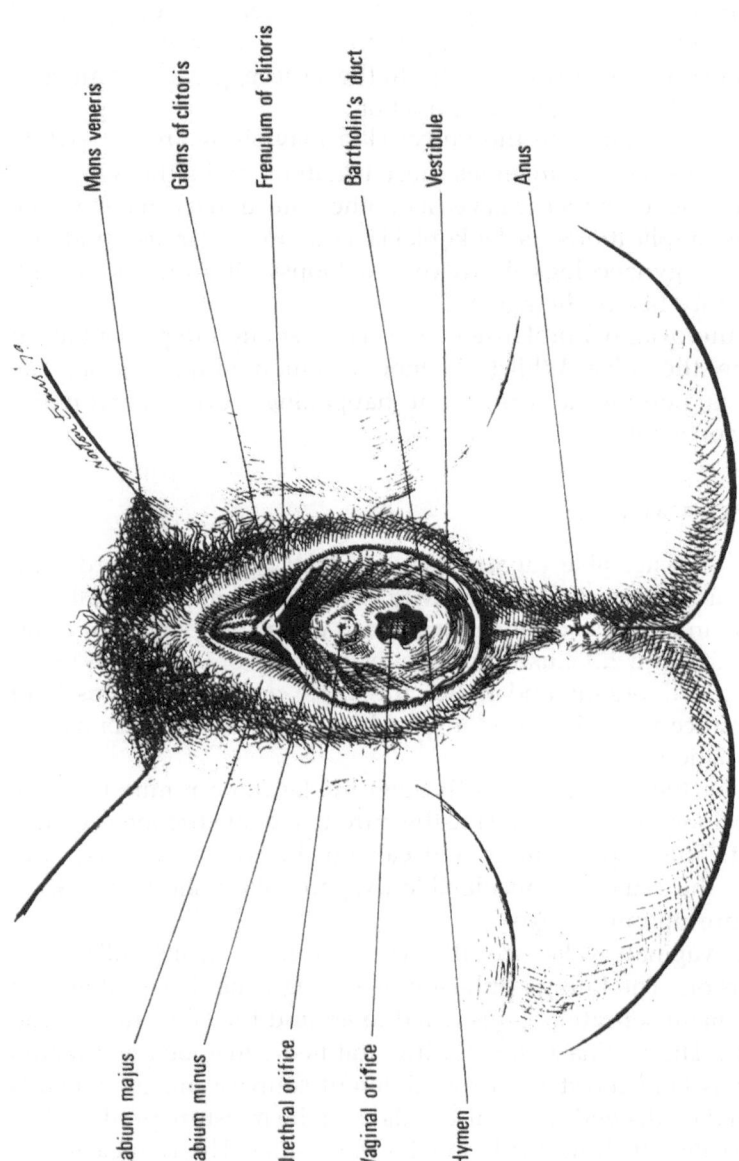

Mons veneris

Glans of clitoris

Frenulum of clitoris

Bartholin's duct

Vestibule

Anus

Labium majus

Labium minus

Urethral orifice

Vaginal orifice

Hymen

Figure 2.1 External appearance of the female.

On either side of the vagina are special erectile muscles, the corpora cavernosa, and these become engorged during sexual foreplay in readiness for coital penetration. In view of this delicate and sensitive area being so close to the surface, great care must be exercised during vaginal examination.

With increasing age the vulval skin may show areas of white plaque which can sometimes cause irritation, and although this is usually due to a superficial yeast or other infection it can have more sinister implications as leukoplakia is a precancerous condition requiring gynaecological advice and biopsy. It would be a rare occurrence before the age of 55.

An uterovaginal prolapse may be large enough to present at, or outside, the vulva. Whilst it is more common with increasing age there is nothing to prevent it happening during a woman's reproductive life.

2.2 THE VAGINA

This is a distensible tubal structure which extends upwards and backwards towards the concavity of the sacrum. The walls are usually in such close contact with each other that they form a slit. Look at Figure 2.2 illustrating the relationship of the vagina to the other pelvic organs and notice the angle described as this is of importance when inserting a speculum or performing a bimanual examination.

Where the vagina passes through the levator ani muscle of the pelvic floor, about 2 cm inside the introitus, a constriction ring may be felt. This is particularly noticeable if the woman is tense, and can be the cause of considerable dyspareunia if she is unable to relax during intercourse.

The vaginal walls are thrown into folds which allow for distension. The lining epithelium is not particularly sensitive and in the main sensation is restricted to around the labia minora and clitoris. The vagina is lined with stratified squamous epithelium which is kept moist from two different sources; mucus which is secreted by the endocervical glands, and the moisture produced by lactobacilli which normally inhabit the vagina. The lactobacilli are known as Döderlein's bacilli; they digest glycogen in the cervical secretion and the most superficial vaginal cells, and while this is going on they form water and lactic acid. In this way the vagina is kept clear of pathogens which cannot survive in the acid

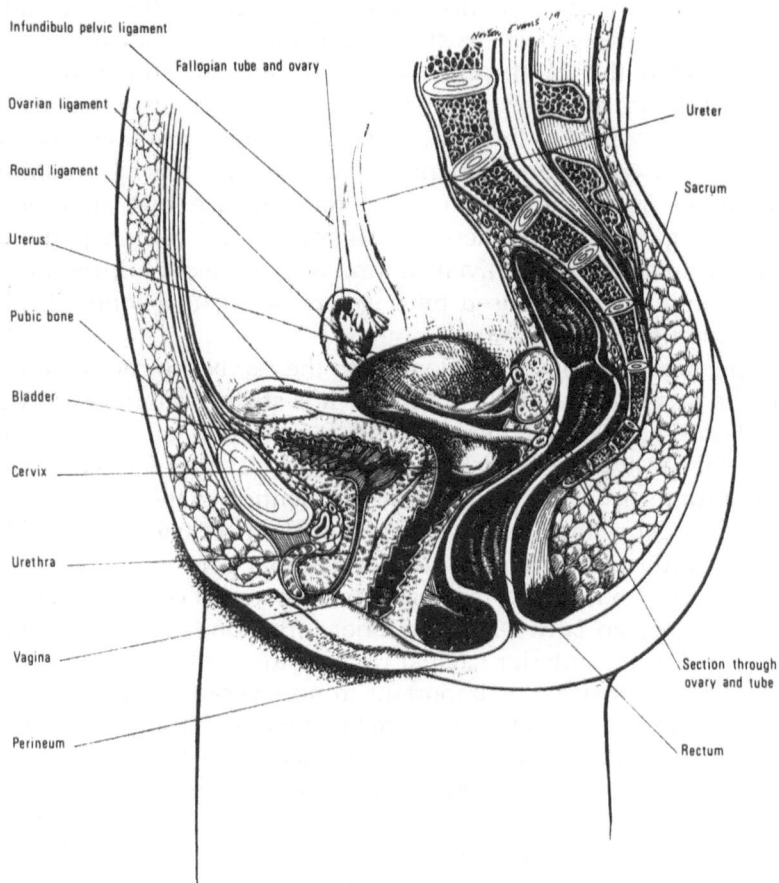

Infundibulo pelvic ligament

Fallopian tube and ovary

Ovarian ligament

Round ligament

Uterus

Pubic bone

Bladder

Cervix

Urethra

Vagina

Perineum

Ureter

Sacrum

Section through ovary and tube

Rectum

Figure 2.2 Sagittal section of the female pelvis.

environment (pH 4–4.5). However, the balance may be upset if the bacilli are killed by a course of antibiotics intended for a systemic infection elsewhere. The acidity can also be altered by the contraceptive pill, over-fastidious attention to personal hygiene and the use of sprays, deodorants and highly scented toiletries: in these cases it is quite probable that yeasts such as monilia will flourish.

Some lubrication is provided during the pre-coital excitement by two Bartholin's glands, situated on either side of the vaginal orifice about 1.5 cm above the fourchette. Only the ducts can be seen, as the glands are situated deep within the erectile tissue already described. Occasionally blockage of a duct can result in painful distension of the gland, particularly if the mucoid contents become infected, and in these cases surgical drainage is essential with, wherever possible, retention of the gland. This operation is called marsupialization. Family planning staff will see this very painful condition from time to time and must realize that an urgent surgical opinion may be necessary although some doctors prefer to try and treat it conservatively at first, with antibiotics. Infection of the glands may be caused by a variety of organisms but chiefly gonococcus or *Escherichia coli*.

The vagina is about 8 cm long with the cervix protruding in the upper part of the anterior wall, which is slightly shorter than the posterior wall. A circular channel can be defined around the cervical protrusion which is described as the fornices. The posterior fornix is worthy of particular mention as this is where the semen is deposited and it is essential that an occlusive diaphragm fits correctly and comfortably into this upper part of the vagina. If the diaphragm is not correctly inserted it may not cover the cervix, but rest instead between the anterior fornix and the pubic bone. Adjacent to the anterior vaginal wall are the bladder and urethra. Their close proximity is important to note because if the bladder remains unemptied before examination for a cap fitting it can cause discomfort and worse, result in an inaccurate fitting. It is the nurse's responsibility to remind each woman to empty her bladder before examination.

The vaginal epithelium covers a thin layer of loose connective tissue and surrounding this are circular and longitudinal pelvic floor muscles (Figure 2.3). If these become overstretched during child-birth, prolapse of the bladder (cystocoele) or rectum (rectocoele) may be seen or felt either on direct examination or when the woman is asked to cough or strain. Weakness of the ligaments, especially the two cardinal ligaments which are situated to either side of the cervix, will be evident by prolapse of the uterus and cervix which is known as vault prolapse. Any laxity in the vaginal musculature or weakness of the pelvic floor muscles may make female barrier methods of contraception unsatisfactory. Prolapse is also noteworthy as some women will seek advice and reassurance about 'something coming down', bladder or bowel symptoms or even bleeding from traumatic ulceration of the protruding lump. Older women may on occasion be too embarrassed to seek advice

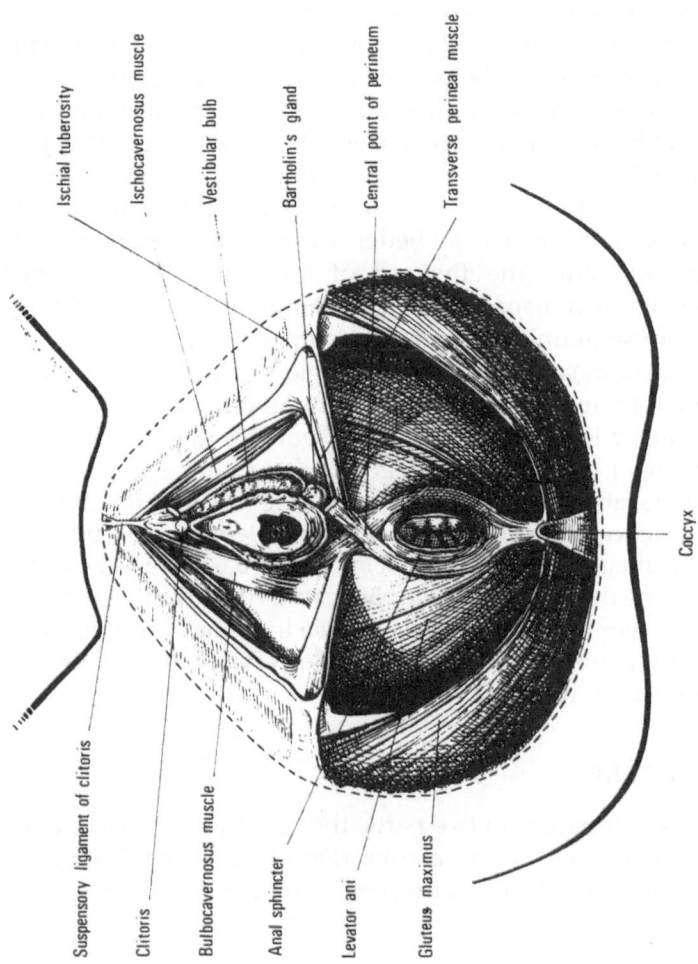

Ischial tuberosity

Ischocavernosus muscle

Vestibular bulb

Bartholin's gland

Central point of perineum

Transverse perineal muscle

Coccyx

Suspensory ligament of clitoris

Clitoris

Bulbocavernosus muscle

Anal sphincter

Levator ani

Gluteus maximus

Figure 2.3 Muscular section of the female external genitalia and pelvic floor.

from their general practitioner, preferring to mention their anxieties in a clinic.

The hymen is a thin ring of tissue perforated in the centre or in several places to permit drainage of menstrual blood. Whilst it is traditional to associate the intact hymen with virginity the widespread use of menstrual tampons means that in many women the hymen is stretched before intercourse can cause rupture. In some cases rupture of the hymen during the honeymoon with evidence of bleeding is an essential event for proof of both the girl's virginity and consummation of the marriage. It is most essential that the wishes of those women who are part of this culture should be respected and it is usually better if vaginal examination can be deferred until after the first act of intercourse has occurred. Occasionally an unusually tough or minutely perforated hymen can cause dyspareunia (painful intercourse) or apareunia (inability to perform coitus) and may require surgical incision. A completely imperforate hymen will usually present as primary amenorrhoea or occasionally lower abdominal pain, but this might be expected in the younger girl around the age of menarche.

Congenital abnormalities of the vagina are rare findings at family planning clinics, but occasionally a vaginal septum may be found as either a small band or a complete double-barrelled vagina. It is caused by the developmental duplication of the lower genital tract during embryonic life which fails to fuse into one, and this sort of abnormality may also result in a double cervix with or without a double uterus as well.

2.3 THE UTERUS

The uterus is described in two parts, the cervix and the body of the uterus, also known as the corpus (Figures 2.4 and 2.5). These together measure 7–8 cm and resemble an inverted pear.

The cervix

The cervix is the lower one third of the uterus. Part of the cervix protrudes through the anterior wall of the vagina at the upper end and can be seen on speculum examination as a smooth shiny knob which is distinct from the convoluted vaginal wall. The size of the vaginal portion of the cervix depends on the woman's parity. It is about 2 cm in diameter in women who have never had a child, and

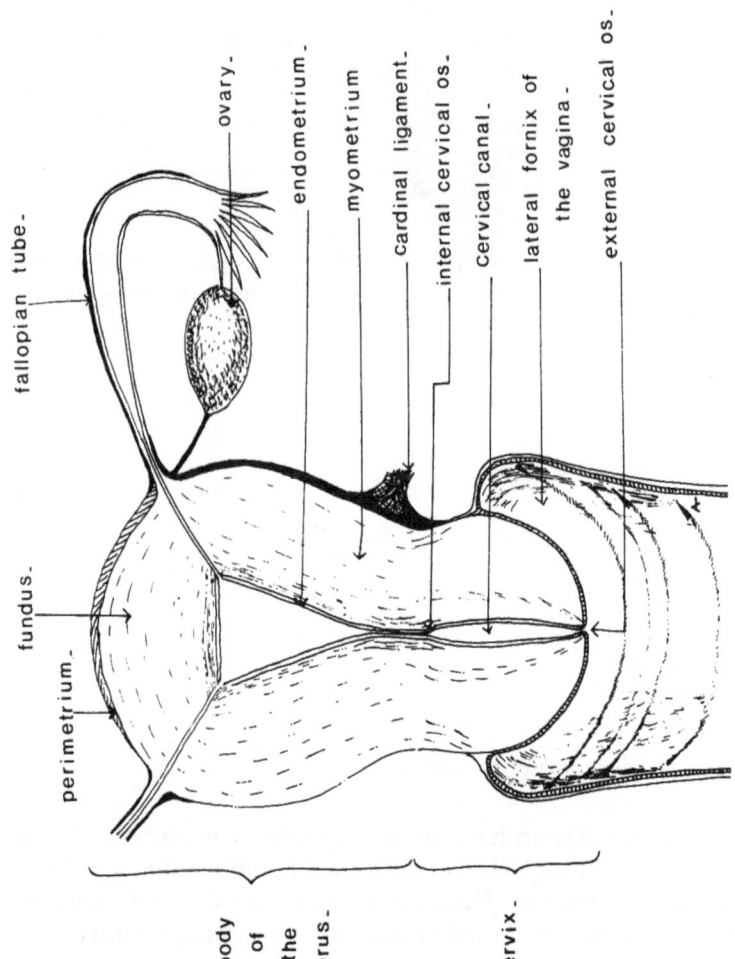

Figure 2.4 Anatomy of the uterus.

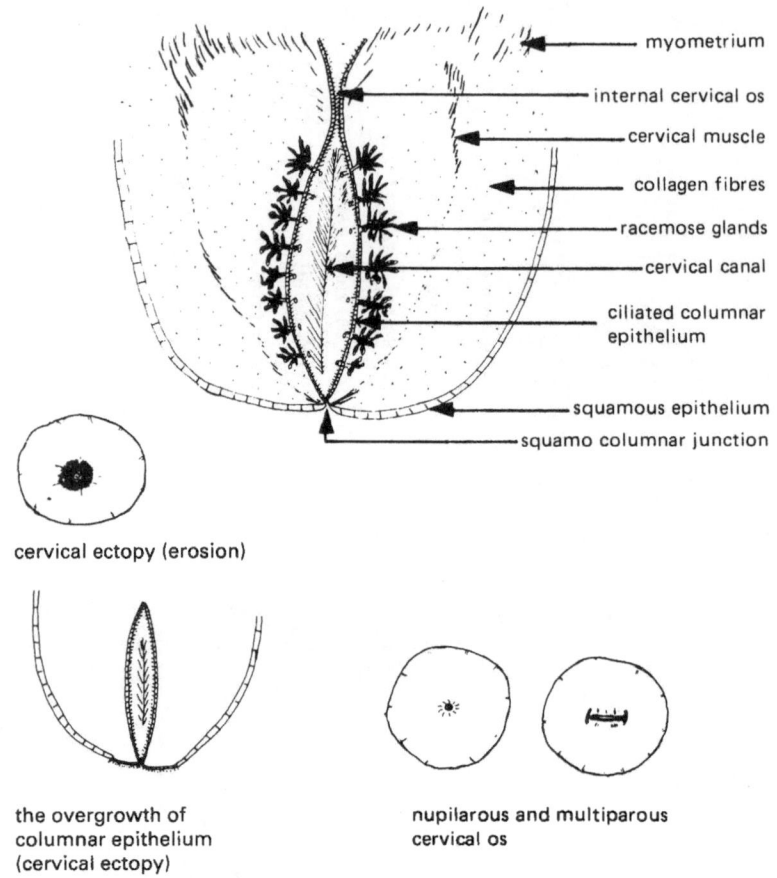

myometrium

internal cervical os

cervical muscle

collagen fibres

racemose glands

cervical canal

ciliated columnar epithelium

squamous epithelium

squamo columnar junction

cervical ectopy (erosion)

the overgrowth of columnar epithelium (cervical ectopy)

nupilarous and multiparous cervical os

Figure 2.5 The anatomy of the cervix.

will be larger if children have been delivered. The entrance to the uterine cavity is through the cervical canal and the outer opening is known as the external os. This appears as a central dimple in primiparous women, but after vaginal delivery it has the appearance of a horizontal slit.

The cervix consists mainly of collagen fibres within which there is a small but none-the-less important ring of muscle at the upper end of the cervical canal forming the internal cervical os where the uterine cavity begins. Miscarriages and premature labour may sometimes occur because of a weakness of the internal os, and continued retention of an IUD also depends on good function of this muscle.

At the external os the squamous epithelium, which covers the vagina and the external portion of the cervix, meets the columnar epithelium which lines the cervical canal and the uterine cavity. The two skin types are in delicate equilibrium, but overactivity of the columnar cells can sometimes occur at the expense of the squamous cells which results in the gross appearance known as ectopy. This can be seen when using a speculum as a red velvety lesion surrounding the external os. The cells which are usually protected within the canal are open to damage and infection and although many cervical erosions are asymptomatic and a chance finding, a small number cause vaginal discharge. The squamo–columnar junction is the area from which cervical smears (Pap Smears) are taken because it is the area of maximum cellular activity. If the smear is normal and there is no indication for interference nothing further need be done, but where discharge or post-coital bleeding is troublesome, some treatment such as cautery, diathermy or surface freezing by cryosurgery will be necessary. All these treatments leave a raw surface around the squamo–columnar junction which allows fresh re-epithelialization by the correct cell types.

The cavity of the cervix is known as the cervical canal and its walls have deep folds or crypts in the glands of which secretions are produced. These secretions are influenced by the hormonal state of the menstrual cycle. During the pre-ovulatory phase starchy molecules in the cervical mucus are intertwined and form a mesh in which any sperm will be entangled. Then, associated with a surge of oestrogen at ovulation, the physical properties are altered and the previously tenacious and very sticky mucus becomes much more watery as the molecules line up alongside each other in parallel. In this condition the sperm can more easily swim up the lower genital tract like trains speeding along a railway once the points are correctly set, instead of becoming trapped and entangled as a kitten playing, unpermitted, with granny's knitting. Shortly after ovulation the increased progestogen makes the mucus impenetrable once again and it is this effect which is partially responsible for the effectiveness of progesterone-only contraceptives. In this case a physiological sticky plug of cervical mucus remains within the cervix throughout the month.

The body of the uterus

The body of the uterus is covered in a fold of peritoneum on its upper surface, known as the perimetrium. Immediately under this is the thick muscle layer, the myometrium, which forms the bulk of the uterus. The narrow uterine cavity, lined with endometrium, is a continuation of the cervical canal and extends up to the fundus where the fallopian tubes enter. The endometrium undergoes cyclical changes in direct response to circulating levels of the ovarian hormones. Each month the endometrium is shed, and a fresh lining grows from a basal layer to become a thick vascular and glandular bed for a fertilized ovum which is more fully described later (Figure 2.7, p. 20).

The blood supply to the uterus is from both uterine and ovarian arteries, with corresponding venous drainage, which provide a network of vessels capable of hypertrophy during pregnancy when the organ becomes extremely vascular. Occasionally, fibroids develop in the myometrium and whilst these abnormal muscle swellings are benign they may cause heavy periods. Alteration in the pattern of menstrual bleeding or any blood loss from the vagina must be referred for gynaecological opinion. Irregularity around a suspected menopause is no exception to this rule.

2.4 THE FALLOPIAN TUBES

The fallopian tubes (Figure 2.6) enter the uterus bilaterally at the fundus. The two points of entry are called the cornu and from this point they extend for approximately 10 cm in length. This passage in which the sperm fertilizes the ovum varies in width, being very narrow on passing through the myometrium to enter the uterine cavity and gradually widening towards the open, funnel shaped ampulla which has finger-like processes called fimbria. The fimbria help to collect the ovum as it is released from the ovary. The fallopian tube is covered, except for the fimbria, by a reflected fold of peritoneum.

The fallopian tube is designed to collect the ovum released from the ovary at ovulation and convey it to the uterine cavity. During this five day journey the ovum 'expects' to be fertilized, and if intercourse has taken place and sperm have managed to find their way into the tubes they will make contact and fertilization will take place. The fertilized ovum starts developing and dividing whilst it is passing along the tube and it then arrives in the uterine cavity at

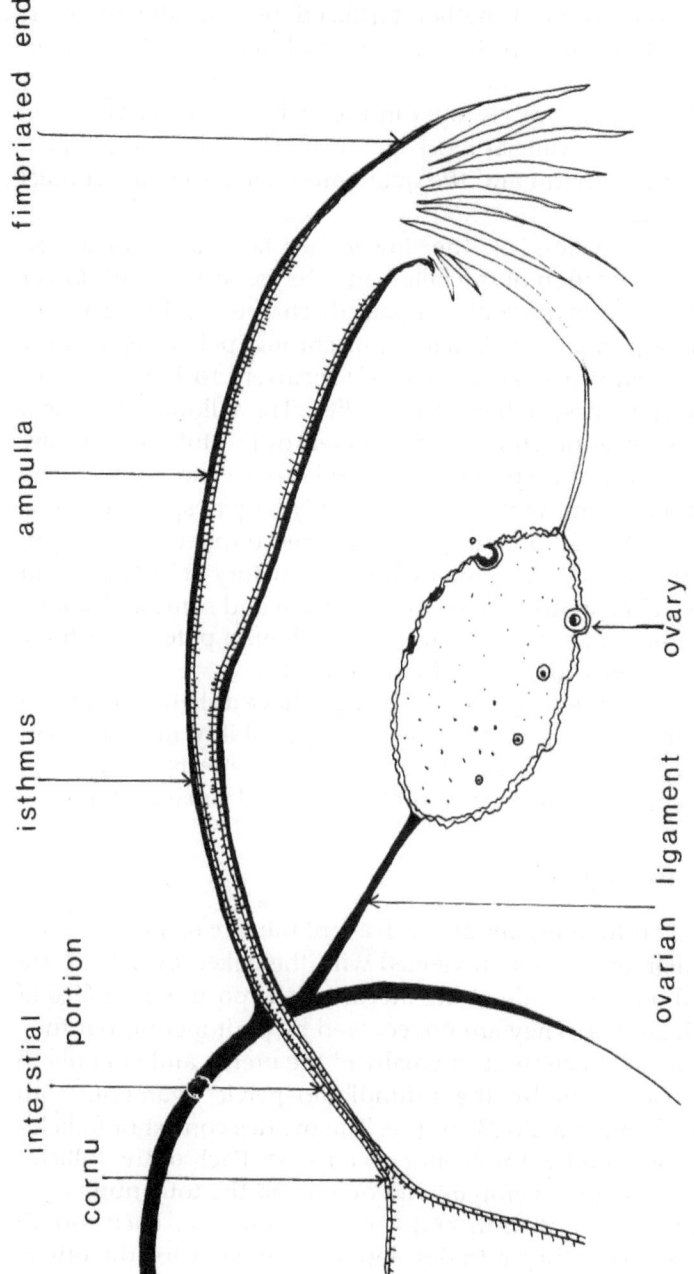

Figure 2.6 Anatomy of the fallopian tubes.

the right stage to be received and commence embedding in the ripened endometrium. Whether fertilized or not, the ovum is wafted along the fallopian tubes by ciliated lining cells. Movement along the tube is also encouraged by peristalsis, which occurs because of a circular muscle layer in the wall. Female sterilization operations rely on artificial blockage or division of both fallopian tubes so that the sperm and the ovum are unable to make contact with each other.

Ascending infection of the lower genital tract can cause salpingitis, an infection of the fallopian tube associated with lower abdominal pain and possible vaginal discharge. Early treatment can eliminate permanent damage, but chronic pelvic sepsis may result in blocked tubes, adhesions and recurrent foci of infection, with the obvious association of infertility. The fallopian tube is a prime target for gonorrhoea. If the lumen of the tube is partially blocked and scarred a sperm may be able to ascend through the system but the ovum, which is considerably larger especially if it is fertilized and already dividing, may become trapped resulting in an ectopic pregnancy. A woman who has a history of infection and presents at a clinic with delayed menstruation and some abdominal discomfort should always be considered to have a potential ectopic pregnancy and has to be seen by the doctor.

Women taking the progestogen-only pill have a slightly increased chance of an ectopic pregnancy and the possibility must be kept in mind. This is because amongst their many effects these preparations seem to utilize an action of diminished tubal motility.

2.5 THE OVARIES

These two glandular organs are each about the size of a walnut and have a similar surface when viewed with the naked eye. They are to be found on either side of the uterus on the posterior surface of the broad ligament. They are not covered by peritoneum, but they have peritoneal attachments medially to the uterus and laterally to the pelvic side wall by the infundibulo–pelvic ligament: both connections contain a blood supply. The ovaries consist of follicles which are contained within connective tissue. Each of the follicles has the potential to develop into an ovum and the total number of follicles are present at birth and cannot regenerate. Each month some of the follicles begin to develop but one outstrips the others and becomes the Graafian follicle from which the ovum will be released at ovulation.

After ovulation the cells remaining in the wall of the follicle change their appearance and become yellow and swollen to form the corpus luteum. This is responsible for providing the hormone progesterone, which is an essential part of the menstrual cycle.

The fimbrial ends of the fallopian tubes are situated close beside the ovaries and are able to move about the surface to catch an ovum once it has been released, so that it may commence its journey along the fallopian tube.

Ovarian cysts may be related to follicles, the corpus luteum, or abnormalities of development. Whilst the majority are benign there is always an underlying risk of ovarian malignancy, so every cyst must be fully investigated by a gynaecologist. With simple cysts it is usually sufficient to shell them out of the ovarian substance thus preserving future function. Whilst one ovary is sufficient for fertility there may be a dominant side and should this be the ovary lost then fertility may be less certain.

2.6 THE MENSTRUAL CYCLE

The menstrual changes generally described as recurring every 28 days are shown in Figure 2.7. Factors influencing the interrelated cycles of the hypothalamus, pituitary, ovary and endometrium are described in the following sections. Each organ is sensitive to the function of related organs and responds to them by a feed-back/cut-off mechanism which balances the rise and fall of hormones as these chemical messengers are released.

The hypothalamic cycle

This cycle initiates the menstrual pattern and originates from the hypothalamus, which is an area situated deep in the brain just above the pituitary gland. It produces a substance which is responsible for stimulating the anterior portion of the pituitary. The hypothalamic cycle can be disturbed by stress and anxiety as well as by alteration of the daily time pattern resulting from long distance air travel. Severe weight loss due to dietary malnutrition or anorexia nervosa may also break the chain resulting in amenorrhoea.

The pituitary gland

The pituitary gland is situated in the base of the skull in a small

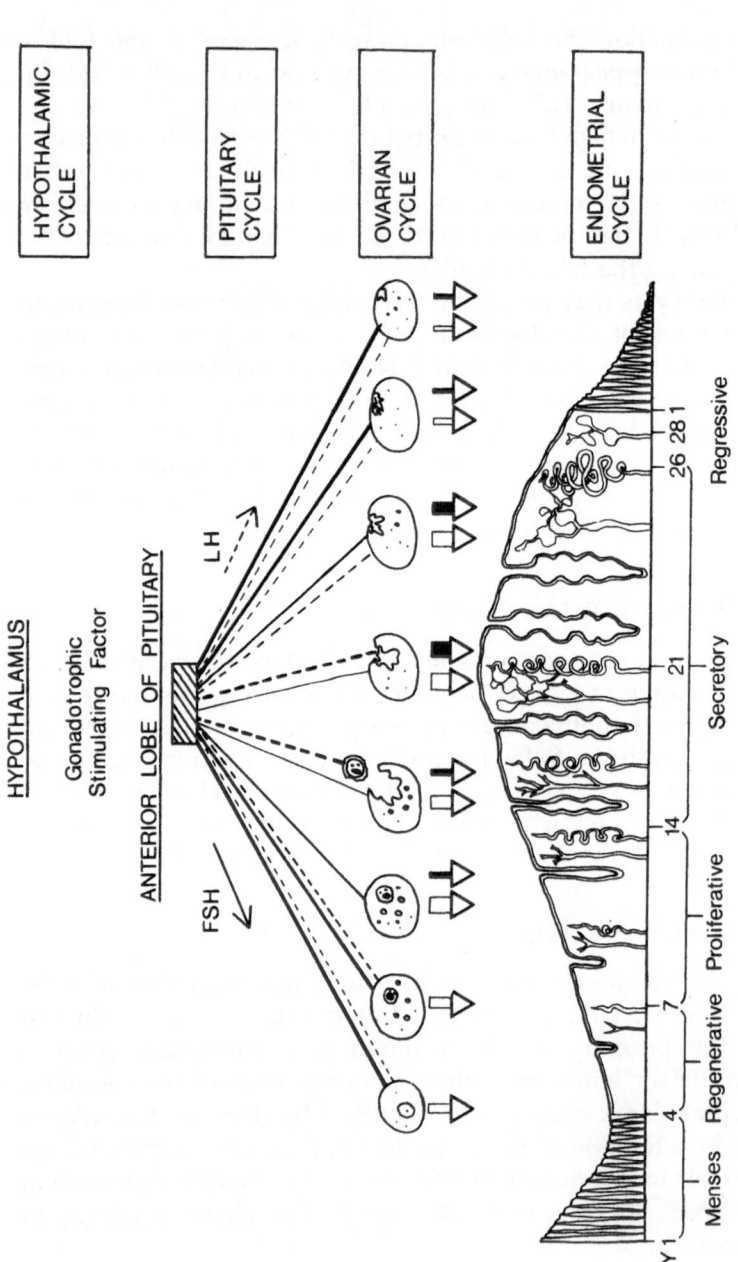

Figure 2.7 The menstrual cycle.

fossa. Only the anterior lobe is influenced by the surrounding hypothalamus which has cyclical control. Amongst several functions the anterior pituitary gland produces follicle stimulating hormone (FSH) and luteinizing hormone (LH) and these two substances stimulate the ovaries to develop follicles and the corpus luteum to ripen.

FSH activates primative follicles in the ovary. Each month several follicles come under the hormonal influence, and a mature ovum ripens. When ovulation has occurred, the pituitary receives information that the event has taken place through high oestrogen levels in the blood. It then reduces the FSH and instead increases LH which assists in maintaining the corpus luteum which is the main source of progesterone during the menstrual cycle.

The ovarian cycle

The follicles within the ovaries are at different stages of maturity and their development is enhanced by regular rises in the amounts of FSH secreted by the pituitary gland. When ripe, the follicle bursts out of its cystic surroundings through the capsular wall of the ovary and is accompanied by some cells and fluid. While the follicle is developing the ovarian tissue is producing oestrogen, a hormone responsible for promoting tissue growth and stimulating secondary sexual characteristics. The oestrogen level rises in the first half of the cycle and is responsible for causing the endometrium to grow and thicken in preparation for the arrival of a fertilized ovum. After ovulation has taken place the cystic space from which the ovum has escaped begins to fill in and heal over and becomes the corpus luteum. The cells lining this crater produce the hormone progesterone, so the level of this hormone is seen to rise in the blood in the second half of the cycle following ovulation. Progesterone stimulates glandular action in the endometrium and causes thickening of the cervical mucus, making it sticky and thus plugging up the cervical canal. At this stage in the cycle the uterus is ready to receive a potential pregnancy. The progesterone raises the basal body temperature slightly, an indication that ovulation has occurred. If no fertilization takes place then the corpus luteum shrivels and the progesterone level falls as a direct result joining diminishing oestrogen which stimulates the pituitary mechanism to start the cycle all over again. The reduction in progesterone also causes the blood supply and glandular action of the endometrium to regress and the endometrial tissue shrinks and becomes anoxic before shedding as menstruation.

The endometrial cycle

The changes occurring in the endometrium are directly due to the influence of ovarian hormones. The first day of menstruation is referred to as day one of the cycle, when the thickened endometrium degenerates and is expelled from the uterus with loss of blood. The menstrual flow varies in quantity and may continue for three to seven days ending with a slight brown discharge. The basal layer of the endometrium remains to grow again, and a short regenerative phase is followed by proliferative growth under the influence of oestrogen.

Following ovulation the increase in progesterone influences the endometrium to become secretory The tortuous glands in the tissue now fatten and produce glycogen and mucus to nourish a fertilized ovum, should it arrive. At this stage the endometrium is very vascular and spongy. Towards the end of the cycle, if no fertilization has taken place, there is a short regressive phase allowing the blood vessels to shrink and reducing the quantity of blood passing through them. Lack of oxygen to the tissue quickly reduces its thickness; it degenerates and is then lost.

It is not uncommon for there to be small variations in cycle length due to the complexity of the interrelated influences. Most women experience some disturbance in the pattern at some time due to emotional stresses or changes in environment and diet. In some cases, as in severe anaemia, starvation or anorexia nervosa, the body, realizing that it cannot afford the stress of pregnancy, will interfere with the cycle and stop menstruation from occurring.

The administration of additional oestrogen and progestogen in the combined pill causes the feedback mechanism in the pituitary to come into action and very little FSH is produced, which in turn prevents ovulation. The balance is a delicate one and women who are unable to take their pills regularly will not only ovulate, but will also suffer from irregular withdrawal bleeding. The levels of oestrogen and progestogen cause endometrial growth to remain rather thin and the delicate tissue bleeds easily but generally much more lightly than a normal period.

3

Male body mechanics

The male reproductive system consists of a pair of testes which are situated within the scrotum; two long ducts (the vas deferens) which convey the sperm formed in the testes to the urethra, and the penis with its special erectile properties necessary for insemination (Figures 3.1 and 3.2). External appearances show the penis and scrotum close together attached to the lower abdomen. However they are connected by a pair of tubal structures known as the vas deferens, one on each side, which pass through the pelvis. This means that the sperm have to make a long journey from the testes where they are produced to the tip of the penis during ejaculation.

3.1 THE SCROTUM

The scrotum is a bag of coarse skin which contains hair follicles and sebaceous glands. Inside is a pair of testes: these originate within the fetal abdomen and are drawn along the inguinal canal by special muscles so that at birth they are present inside the scrotum. The scrotal skin is not attached to the glands, but moves easily over the testes because of a smooth, fluid secreting layer known as the tunica albuginea whose origin lies in the peritoneal pouch brought down with each descending testicle.

The formation of sperm is influenced by temperature, with a high production rate at temperatures slightly lower than normal body heat. It is for this reason that the glands are established inside the scrotum where the temperature is cooler. Regulation is achieved by the cremasteric muscle attached to the upper end of the inner scrotal sac. This muscle can pull the glands closer to the body or allow them to drop further away from the local body heat. The original thermostat for air conditioning!

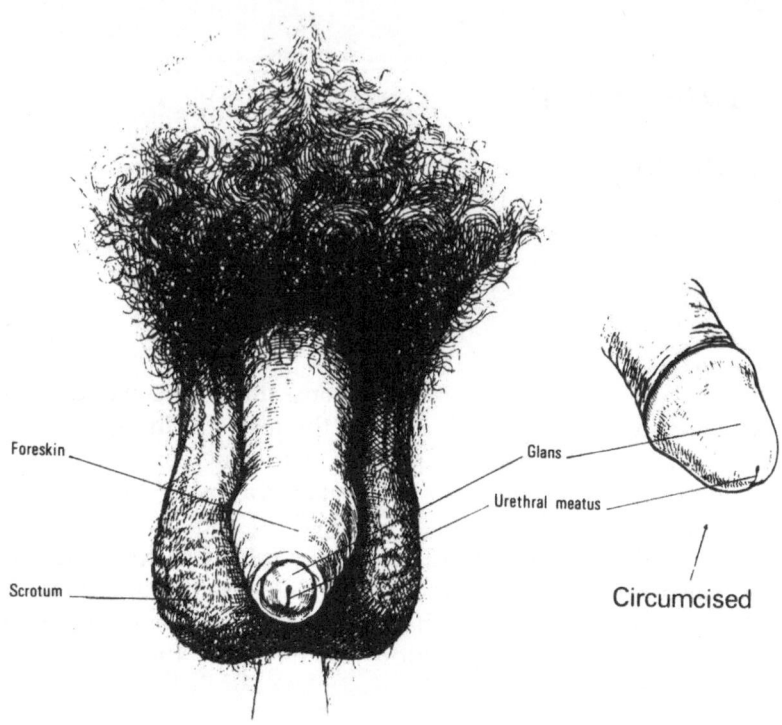

Figure 3.1 External appearance of the male.

3.2 THE TESTES

Each of the bodies felt within the scrotum consists of a testicle and a closely associated coiled structure called the epididymis. Sperm are formed in the testicle and, unlike the ovary, many new sperm cells are being formed continuously. The sperm pass into the epididymis where they mature.

3.3 THE VAS

The vas is a long tubular structure which commences at the lower end of the epididymis and conveys sperm up and out of the scrotum along the inguinal canal to pierce the anterior abdominal wall through the inguinal ring. Once inside, the two vasa are covered with fat and peritoneum and pass on either side of the

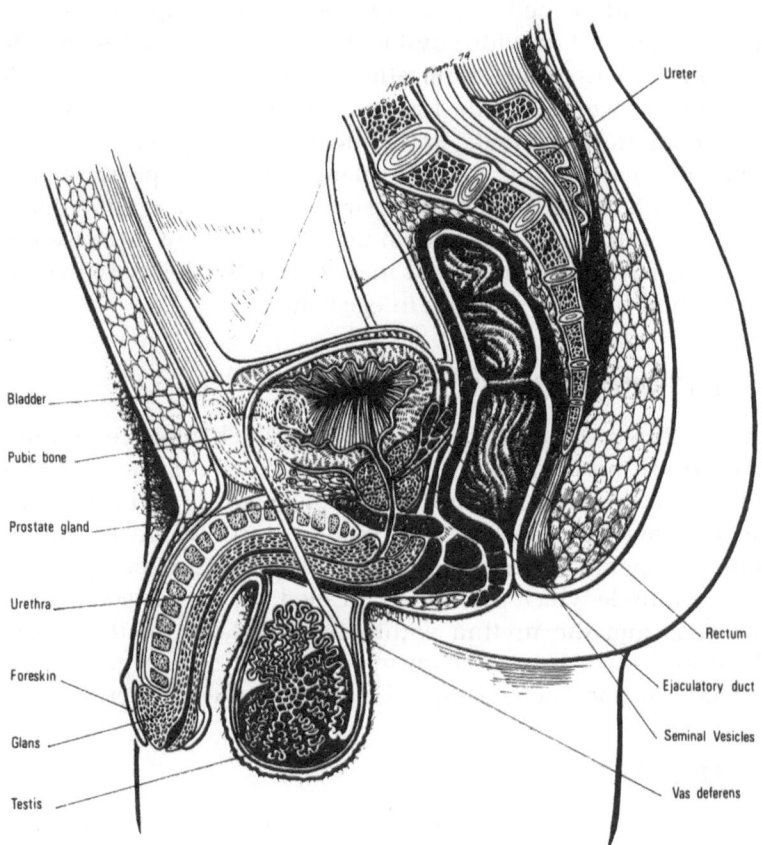

Figure 3.2 Sagittal section of the male pelvis.

bladder before entering the prostate gland which lies beneath it. At this point the vasa connect within two small reservoirs known as seminal vesicles which store mature sperm. Within the prostate gland the two vasa join the membranous urethra forming a single tube for urine from the bladder and semen from the reproductive system.

3.4 THE PROSTATE GLAND

The prostate gland is situated below the bladder base and completely surrounds the urethra. It is responsible for producing prostatic fluid needed to provide energy for the sperm once they are ejaculated. It provides by far the greater part of the ejaculate and this is why male sterilization by vasectomy does not alter apparent function, as the fraction which contains the sperm is small enough not to make any noticeable difference.

Enlargement of the prostate gland with age (prostatitis) can result in retention of urine; this usually requires surgical reduction or removal of the gland, known as prostatectomy. Because of its position, removal of the gland may impair the ability to maintain an erection or cause inability to ejaculate.

3.5 THE URETHRA

The urethra is a dual purpose structure which allows excretion of urine from the bladder and conveys ejaculated semen. The first part of the urethra runs through the pelvic fascia and is known as the membranous urethra. The second part, where the urethra enters the penis, is described as the spongy urethra because of the erectile muscle which surrounds it called the corpus spongiosum. The vasa join the urethra within the substance of the prostate gland and there is a mechanism to prevent semen going in the wrong direction and passing uselessly into the bladder.

3.6 THE PENIS

The penis is a specialized organ which consists of the urethra with its spongy surrounding muscle and a pair of erectile muscles known as the corpora cavernosa. These are placed above the urethra and are contained within a tube of fascia. Erectile tissue works on the principle that if the outflow of blood is restricted, the many venous spaces will fill and become turgid and firm. This capacity for the penis to become erect is controlled by sympathetic and parasympathetic nerves. Whilst essentially a spinal reflex, there is limited higher central nervous control which can initiate or inhibit an erection.

The skin covering the penis is a continuation of the lower abdominal skin. It covers the shaft of the penis and at the outer end a loose fold protects the glans penis. The glans is the external portion of the corpus spongiosum and is covered by very thin and sensitive skin. The protective covering fold of skin is known as the prepuce or foreskin, and may be surgically shortened by the operation of circumcision for religious, ritual or cosmetic purposes, or very occasionally because it is truly tight causing a condition known as phimosis. Where the prepuce is present it is naturally drawn or pushed back during erection or intercourse. A creamy substance may collect under the foreskin and is known as smegma; where this is freely formed, scrupulous attention should be paid to personal hygiene.

The male sexual organs are under the influence of testosterone, the male hormone. They grow and become functional as the amount of this hormone increases at puberty. It influences growth of hair follicles in various parts of the body and this results in beard formation and hair growth in the axilla and pubic areas. Pubic hair is coarse and in adult males extends in a triangle with the apex sometimes as high as the umbilicus. Testosterone also causes the pitch of the male voice to become lower at puberty and this change is heard and described as the 'voice breaking'.

4

The mechanism of
fertilization

4.1 JOURNEY OF SPERM TO EGG

To achieve a pregnancy it is necessary for the sperm to meet and fertilize an ovum travelling through the lumen of the woman's fallopian tube, after which the fertilized ovum continues its journey to the uterine cavity where it is able to settle down and embed itself in the lining layer known as endometrium where it can be nourished and start to grow.

Semen, which contains sperm in a nutrient fluid, is delivered into the lower portion of the female genital tract during the act of intercourse. At copulation the man inserts his erect penis into the woman's vagina which is moist and receptive due to excitatory stimulation. Movement of the penis causes ejaculation and the semen is deposited in the posterior fornix. From there the sperm are attracted to move in the direction of and through the cervical canal, and to some extent this essential step may be assisted by the uterus contracting during orgasm and thereby aspirating some of the semen into the uterine cavity.

The consistency of the mucus plug in the cervical canal is important in deciding whether the sperm can penetrate and make progress through its substance. It has already been described (section 2.3) how the mucus becomes thin and slippery at ovulation when the parallel alignment of the molecules acts rather like setting the points on railway lines to allow the sperm to speed along in the right direction.

Having gained access to the uterine cavity the sperm are attracted by chemotaxis to swim further up the female genital tract in response to chemicals secreted by the zona pelucida of the ovum. The uterine cavity is just a slit as the front and back inner surfaces are pressed together and the sperm move in the thin fluid film by thrusting themselves forward with side to side movements of their flagella or tail. Energy for this propulsive movement is provided by the body of the sperm which metabolizes fructose and other nutrients included in the prostatic fluid which forms most of the ejaculate.

The chemical attraction guides the sperm to the cornua of the uterine cavity and into the lumen of the fallopian tubes where the forward propulsion of the sperm has to overcome a thrust in the opposite direction. This opposing tubal movement is intended to propel the ovum from the open fimbrial end until it reaches the uterus by muscular peristalsis, and this movement is assisted by the lining cells which have microscopic hair-like processes called cilia which waft the egg onwards along the tube. The sperm have therefore to make their way at this stage by running up a down escalator!

4.2 FERTILIZATION

At the lateral free extremity of each fallopian tube a funnel-shaped fimbrial end lies adjacent to an ovary. This end can move to overlie the point where the follicle is developing so that the ovum, when released, may be caught and delivered into the fallopian tube. From there it is moved along the lumen of the tube by the forces described above. Somewhere midway along the fallopian tube the ovum comes into contact with the first of the ascending sperm and is rapidly surrounded by the many sperm which have been attracted to it. It is necessary to have a number of sperm present before one, and one only, manages to penetrate the outer cell membrane and insert its head right into the substance of the ovum. The body and tail then drop off as they are no longer of any use, and the sperm head (containing half the genetic requirements for an embryo) disintegrates to release its half set of chromosomes which are paired with a similar half set already contained in the ovum.

4.3 THE FERTILIZED EGG

With a full complement of chromosomes containing the complete genetic blueprint, the fertilized ovum can start to develop and the original cell is soon duplicating itself by the process of division. Whilst busy dividing and subdividing, the group of cells moves

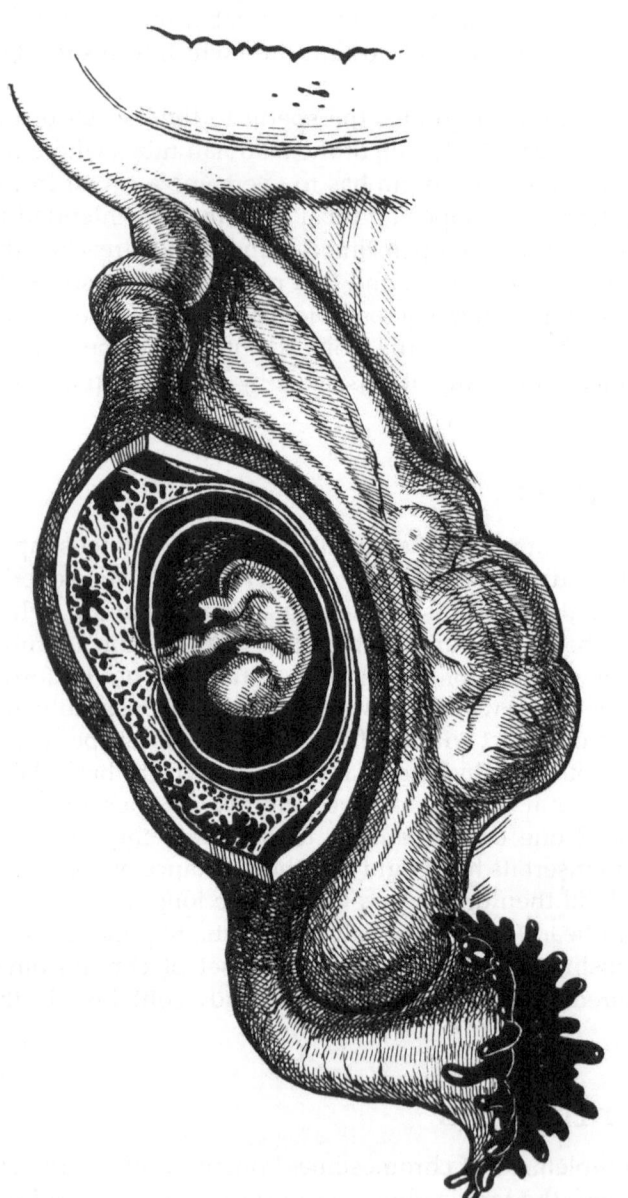

Figure 4.1 Section through tubal pregnancy.

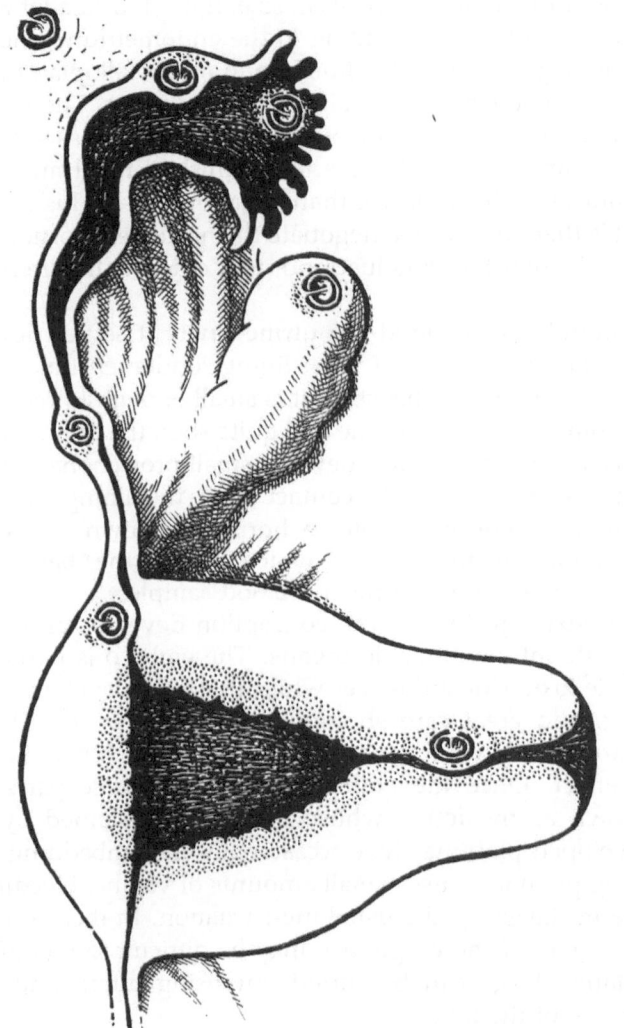

Figure 4.2 Sites of ectopic pregnancy.

along the fallopian tube towards the uterine cavity. The cellular group is known as a morula (a descriptive term coined from the Latin for mulberry!) and it passes through the interstitial part of the tube when it is approximately 12 cells in size. If it is too small it will probably not be ready for embedding in the endometrium, and if any larger it may get stuck in the fine lumen of the fallopian tube and cause an ectopic pregnancy (Figures 4.1 and 4.2). There are suggestions that the increased rate of ectopic pregnancy associated with the use of an IUD may be due to diminished tubal motility causing the morula to have slower than usual progress. This delay means that it is then too large to negotiate the narrowest portion of the fallopian tube which occurs just prior to it entering the uterine cavity.

Once the morula has entered the utrine cavity it settles down within the glandular folds of the lining endometrium and commences embedding. At this stage it is small enough to receive life support from the adjacent tissue and quite soon the outer layer of cells known as the chorion will develop small projections called villi which make more intimate contact with the lining of the endometrium. The chorion secretes a hormone known as HCG (human chorionic gonadotrophin) which forms the basis of pregnancy testing with both urine and blood samples.

During the next eight weeks the conception develops and the cells differentiate into identifiable organs. The embryo is particularly vulnerable to outside influences whilst this basic development is proceeding, and great care should be shown with regard to prescribing drugs and avoiding certain infections which may have an adverse effect. Once the embryo has all the basic parts it becomes known as the fetus, whose growth is sustained by a properly developed placenta. Just occasionally the embedding of the developing placenta causes small amounts of vaginal bleeding which can be mistaken for the usual menstruation. In these cases the commencement of the pregnancy may be difficult to identify, but the gestational age can be sorted out using ultrasound to measure the size of the fetus.

Following the initial cellular upheavals demanded by the development of the embryo and its specialized organ requirements, the fetus grows on steadily from 12 weeks without any further major design changes until it is ready to be born and live independently of its mother, about 38 weeks after fertilization took place. (This is calculated as 40 weeks after the last normal menstrual period assuming that the mother has a 28 day menstrual cycle.)

5

Clinic organization

The Department of Health provides general guidelines on health provision and controls the total funding available for each Regional Health Authority (RHA). The RHA is at the top of the administrative structure of the National Health Service (NHS) and controls the finance available to each District Health Authority (DHA). It is up to the District General Manager to provide effective family planning and well-woman services. Many family doctors have been trained in the required skills and are undertaking increasing responsibility for this primary health-care service. In most practices the primary health care team includes practice nurses who have been trained on the ENB course 900/901.

The family planning service is not the exclusive province of the NHS. There are some independent organizations which offer the service, and there are a few clinics which due to quirks within the NHS arrangements still come under the administration of their own governing bodies or contract with the DHA for the service. For example, the Family Planning Association (FPA) may run their own service for the benefit of the District medical services. In the past most of the family planning clinics were provided by the FPA under contractual agreements with local authorities, but following the reorganization of the NHS in 1974 these clinics became the responsibility of the DHAs who most commonly took over the management of staff resources and premises.

The aim of family planning is to provide advice and contraception, often within the NHS, to anyone who requests it. In order to do this work efficiently it is necessary to use all premises to their best advantage. The facilities may be modern, purpose built units, but very many are still in converted houses or sections of cottage-type hospitals. There is little alteration which can be made to the interior of old buildings for economic reasons, but with ingenuity, available accommodation may be adapted to good use.

5.1 ACCESS AND APPOINTMENTS SYSTEM

Clinic premises should be easily accessible to clients, and the entrance wide enough to admit prams and wheelchairs, with space provided indoors for their 'parking'. The lack of direct public transport and car parking facilities are obviously great disadvantages.

The prime need in clinics is the introduction of a sound appointments system, and every effort should be made to adhere to the times as this contributes greatly to the smooth running of the clinic by reducing the waiting times to a minimum, and brings a welcome degree of order for the staff. Some undesignated spare time needs to be included in the timetable to absorb the casual attender who may urgently need to be seen. In some centres it seems to be more acceptable to have a walk-in session which may be particularly useful for the younger age group. All staff must be aware that no one should be sent away without recourse to nursing or medical advice.

5.2 WAITING AREAS AND TOILET FACILITIES

The waiting area must be able to accommodate more than the expected number of people who usually attend in case staff shortage causes delay. An ample supply of suitable literature is recommended for those waiting, and contraceptive and health education pamphlets should be attractively displayed and available for people to read and take away.

A great deal of time can be saved if a prominent notice is displayed as a reminder that the date of the last normal menstrual period will be requested at each attendance. Another helpful prompt concerns those seeking a pregnancy test who should either have brought an early morning specimen of urine or be prepared to provide a sample for testing.

Good toilet facilities must be available in all clinics and they should be supervised by a member of the clinic staff.

5.3 RECEPTION AND DISPENSING AREAS

These areas, which often have multipurpose use, should aim to be shielded from the waiting area in order to increase the degree of privacy. There should be ease of access for the reception clerks to handle case notes, general records and registers: telephones which will need to be constantly answered must be within easy reach. If it is also a dispensing area sufficient space must be available for contraceptive stores.

The clerical staff and receptionists have a very important part to play in establishing a friendly atmosphere in the clinic. They are the first to greet people when they arrive and should be able to make them feel at home. Contraceptive services are used by both men and women so it is important that they are given equal encouragement to request advice. The creation of friendly and co-operative relationships between the clerical and clinical staff will stimulate the development of a good team spirit which will provide strength in times of stress. Every encouragement should be given to the clerical support staff to work with enthusiasm and assurance; a little appreciation of their efforts on the 'front line' never goes astray.

5.4 CONSULTATION, EXAMINATION AND WAITING ROOMS

These rooms need to be quiet, warm, well lit and ventilated. Where possible they should be large enough to contain an examination couch and other necessary furniture. An adjustable examination lamp capable of providing strong directional illumination is essential. Rooms should be prepared in advance with an adequate supply of appropriate sterile equipment. Great emphasis should be placed on privacy and cleanliness. People requesting contraception need to talk in private with a nurse or doctor without any disturbance or interruption. Facilities for undressing should be considered with easy access to toilets. Changing rooms and couches should be kept clean and fresh, with an ample supply of clean linen and paper so that the couch covers can be changed for each person.

5.5 STERILE EQUIPMENT

A considerable amount of equipment is now disposable or supplied in sterile packs and this has improved speed and efficiency. Packs are supplied from the local hospital sterile supply department (CSSD) and will remain sterile until opened unless the wrapping is damaged. This system entirely depends on a regular delivery and on careful return of used items for reprocessing, both of which require responsible management. Equipment which has been used should be carefully collected and returned without rinsing in the appropriate containers provided. The replacement of lost or damaged equipment is very expensive and every precaution should be taken to avoid such losses and the expenditure incurred.

Occasionally, staff may need to resort to sterilizing on the premises and small portable autoclaves are available which only need to be plugged in to a normal electric power point. In less ideal circumstances clean instruments can be soaked in activated gluteraldehyde (Cidex) which will kill off most organisms in ten minutes (although more persistent spores may require immersion for three hours). It is vital that the object is totally immersed, and thoroughly rinsed before use. In emergencies instruments can be sterilized by immersing them for two minutes in a 0.5% solution of chlorhixidine gluconate (Hibitaine) in 70% alcohol and then rinsing with sterile water.

5.6 SPECIMENS

Arrangements for obtaining cytological smears and bacteriological swabs, accurate labelling and matching with completed request forms are the responsibility of the clinical staff. The final collection of specimens should be checked and recorded in a book so that results can be noted, recalled easily and any delay investigated.

5.7 PREGNANCY TESTING

Pregnancy testing is part of the clinic service and the equipment should be kept in a refrigerator or a cool place when not in use. Some clinics do not, as yet, have their own equipment and are obliged to send the specimen to the local hospital for testing which results in several additional days of anxious waiting. However, with simple, cheap and certain methods readily available this should now be unnecessary.

5.8 STORES

A good supply of all contraceptives in regular use should be kept in stock. The quantities kept in store need constant assessment and reordering to maintain the supply. Overstocking of infrequently used items must be avoided to prevent wastage. All stocks should be secured under lock and key and should have ample space so that all contraceptives are stored in an orderly fashion. A supply of pamphlets for all the contraceptive methods also needs to be kept. Useful teaching aids may also require space in the cupboard. In addition there should be a number of small teaching boxes containing a variety of caps, IUDs and pills for the convenience of each clinician.

It is wise to have some other medications such as mild analgesia available, and a small stock of antibiotics which may be prescribed during evening clinic sessions.

5.9 RECORDS

An outline of what was discussed, requested, advised and implemented should be clearly written in each case record at every visit to the clinic. Records of blood pressure, weight and the date of the last normal menstrual period should be indicated where appropriate. Results of any tests should be inserted on return and checked by a doctor or nurse. As a legal document these case notes are an *aide-mémoire*, and proof that the individual has received a full explanation about the chosen method, how to use it, and its possible dangers and side effects. When the nurse has dealt with teaching the method to the woman, an entry should be made to this effect. If extra pages are added they should have the name and clinic number of the woman written on them. The general practitioner should, when the person agrees, be notified of the action being advised by the clinic and, where necessary, his advice regarding the suitability of the chosen contraceptive should be sought.

Confidentiality of these records is of the utmost importance, and legitimate complaints can be made if this confidentiality is breached. It should also be remembered that under the Data Protection Act individuals have the legal right to view information stored about themselves, and notes should always be compiled with this in mind. There are usually well established retrieval systems for storing case records, and there should be cross-reference cards kept separately with the name, address, date of birth and registration number recorded, as some people are bound to arrive without their appointment card bearing the case note number. Changes of name and address should be attended to at once and noted at each appropriate place in the records.

The next appointment is made at the end of the clinic visit. Timely reminders about keeping appointments and collecting all belongings before departure may assist future clinic arrangements, and should help to reduce the pile of lost umbrellas and children's toys which come to light when everybody has gone home.

5.10 STAFF MEETINGS

Regular meetings between all members of the staff should be arranged, and doctors and nurses who may only work for a few sessions should be welcome to attend. These meetings are valuable for bringing new developments to everybody's notice. They are particularly valuable in clinics isolated from hospital centres, where staff have to rely on fragile and impersonal methods of communication with doctors and laboratory technicians dealing with referrals. It is also an ideal opportunity for meeting people socially from other service departments on whom the clinic staff rely, so that any problem that arises from time to time can be sorted out at a personal level and positive improvements made. Sometimes these meetings can have an educational element by arranging to invite a guest speaker to talk on an interesting aspect of contraception, and this form of enlivenment may encourage those who find the more formal meeting unattractive.

6

The first clinic visit

A wide variety of individuals seek advice about contraception. Many of these choose to attend a family planning clinic and first impressions will be very important to them. They are seeking expert advice and help with a personal situation which they wish to control. How far their planning succeeds depends on intelligence, luck and the quality of the professional advice given. Doctors and nurses at the clinic have a special role to play in the success of creating the right atmosphere of ease and friendliness in which people seeking contraceptive advice can gain confidence. Nobody interested in people can resist the rich variety of personalities which every clinic brings. Whilst some women will arrive with a clear idea about what method of contraception suits them, others will be less certain and need an outline of all the available methods; yet others will attend with problems less clearly associated to contraception. Clinic staff therefore need to have much patience, sensitivity and, above all, insight to deal with all of them successfully.

It must be stressed that most qualified nurses and doctors on family planning courses will need to adopt a fresh attitude altogether in their approach to people attending family planning clinics. This is made easier if it is remembered that clinic staff are no longer dealing with patients compelled by illness to seek care, and there is no requirement for someone to act with authority in taking decisions for them. Staff will often find themselves used as sounding boards for people unravelling their problems, and so comes the need to cultivate the role of an understanding friend with expertise to help them make their own correct decisions. Although women make up the bulk of clinic visitors and are consequently referred to most often, men also attend, accompanying their wives or partners and occasionally on their own. Many immigrant couples come together and it is quite usual for the husband to take responsibility for translating and explaining the dialogue on these occasions.

A good appointments system is a great help in the smooth running of a family planning clinic and a realistically adequate amount of time should be allocated to first visits to ensure that a full and correct history and examination along with discussion and teaching of the chosen method can be undertaken. A build-up of pressure on time causes much frustration and harassment, both to clinic personnel and to those waiting to be seen, and this should be avoided.

6.1 INTERVIEWING SKILLS

Obtaining a concise history requires considerable skill. During the course of general nurse training the histories of patients are usually obtained by doctors and medical students and many a nurse's skill in this field is poorly developed. Implementation of the nursing process to training schools will hopefully rectify this to some degree. Postgraduate courses in Midwifery or Health Visiting give opportunities to carry out history taking. However, the experience will be new for some nurses, and guidance and support will be necessary. Part of the secret to be learnt comes from the attitude of the individual nurse and her ability to put people completely at their ease.

It is important to stress again that at these interviews the person attending the clinic does so voluntarily and is not a patient with an illness. Every nurse training in family planning, perhaps more especially those who are well qualified and holding more senior appointments, could benefit from careful personal reappraisal, and should welcome advice on changing the manner of approach from that of authority and efficiency to a more relaxed, friendly and attentive attitude. An authoritarian attitude may be so strongly developed that any inhibition goes unrecognized. There is no need to fear that exposure of a more gentle nature will make a nurse more vulnerable and less capable: indeed, it will make her much more approachable and acceptable to everyone attending the clinic.

The ability to conduct an interview well is very largely dependent on establishing a comfortable atmosphere. Ideally, the interview should be conducted in a quiet, warm and well ventilated room, adequately lit and furnished so that those involved can converse with each other quite informally in privacy and without fear of interruption. Unfortunately, clinic premises vary considerably in the facilities they provide and staff must be encouraged to adapt the existing environment to the best possible advantage. In some clinics the premises are far from ideal and interviews may have to be conducted in the corner of a crowded waiting room or in a busy passage. It then becomes even more essential for the nurse to develop a close rapport with the woman by concentrating her attention so directly on her that she soon becomes unaware of the presence of everyone else. This is facilitated if the woman is seated facing the nurse and with her back to the crowd.

One of the purposes of the interview is to discover any contraindications to the various forms of contraception, in order to prevent problems. The contraindications are dealt with in the appropriate chapters describing the various methods but some are briefly mentioned here to illustrate how they can be perceived in the interview situation. Those taking histories must develop a sense of heightened awareness, and not only listen carefully to a woman's replies, but also have the ability to observe signs of anxiety often expressed in non-verbal ways. Awareness of what is not said is insufficiently developed in nurse and medical training and is largely underestimated in the early professional years. If the nurse finds that the woman has disclosed some particular anxiety, then opportunity should be given for her to explore it further. It should never be cut short by dismissing it lightly with meaningless reassurances.

If the nurse is to feel free to give her whole attention to the interview, it becomes essential that she should make herself familiar beforehand with the details of the information she requires and with the different types of notes provided by the clinic. She should also listen critically during the interview and note additional information offered which may need further investigation. In that way nothing important will be missed.

6.2 DETAILS REQUIRED AT THE INTERVIEW

The nurse should ask the woman at the beginning of the interview what she feels the clinic can do for her and, according to her reply, begin to note the information she must obtain by adapting, as necessary, the order of the questions given below for guidance. The explanatory notes added to the details required indicate the motives that lie behind the questions!

Name and address

It is important to write the first names, surname and address on the record sheet and folder so that the woman can be contacted if necessary after she leaves the clinic. Always confirm that it will be acceptable for the clinic to use the address without embarrassment.

Age

This information may be relevant if oral contraception is requested. Sometimes women with anxieties about the menopause come to the clinic to seek advice. Occasionally, girls who are under the legal age of consent of 16 years come to the clinic seeking help: they need to be specially advised (section 14.1).

Smoker or non-smoker

This is relevant, with other factors, if oral contraception is requested because smoking increases the mortality and morbidity.

Name and address of general practitioner

The general practitioner should be notified if oral contraception is prescribed or if the woman is fitted with an IUD (intrauterine device). It is also important to keep the doctor informed of the results of any pathological investigations. The woman should be told that the clinic will normally notify her own family doctor, and if she expresses concern, it should be discussed with the clinic doctor.

Employment or training

It is useful to ask for this information in order to be able to offer advice on contraceptive methods in an acceptable way. It should never be assumed that a person does not require careful advice because of her background, or previous use or familiarity with methods of contraception. It is, for example, easy to assume that medical and nursing professionals know what to do and can manage for themselves but this may be far from the truth and they may be too embarrassed to admit their ignorance and hurry off without the help which they would have received had it been tactfully offered. Women whose work involves a lot of travel need to have flexible arrangements made for prescriptions and future visits. Difficulties and tensions which arise from unemployment should this be mentioned, may sometimes be helpfully discussed.

Marital state

It is best if the full names as well as the surname are written on the cover of the notes as it avoids the prefix 'Mrs' or 'Miss' when calling the woman. It is helpful however to know whether relationships are permanent, indefinite or temporary as each group has its own stresses and strengths which may affect the attitude to a particular method of contraception. Knowledge of the woman's and/or partner's employment allows for a more accurate assessment of the family lifestyle. For instance, a husband whose job takes him away from home irregularly will not find adapting to 'the safe period' very rewarding.

Previous methods of birth control

Some useful information should emerge from a brief discussion of previous methods, such as the length of time that the woman has been using contraception and also any difficulties that have arisen. Women will seldom wish to resume a previously unsatisfactory method and careful attention during discussion may provide clues that will help the nurse to discover the couples who are experiencing problems with intercourse. These people need quiet encouragement to discuss the matter with a doctor or nurse experienced in psychosexual counselling.

If no contraception has been used it is worth enquiring if they have had unprotected intercourse in case pregnancy has occurred. It is also helpful to know whether intercourse has even been attempted so that examining the woman can be delayed until a later visit and the doctor duly briefed.

Menstrual history

Clear details are essential before any method of contraception can be discussed. The length of the menstrual cycle and its regularity, quantity and quality of blood loss since the menarche should be noted. Any missed periods or variation of the cycle will be important for the doctor to know about when selecting a suitable oral contraceptive. The date of onset of the last period should be stated and any hesitancy in the reply followed up to ensure that there is no chance of any pregnancy having occurred.

Abnormalities of menstrual bleeding
If the woman has always had a scant blood loss, or if she is very young and has not established regular periods, it may be unwise to consider oral contraception.

Menorrhagia, when the quantity of blood lost is heavy, may initially be difficult to establish. In an attempt to gauge the actual blood lost it is helpful to ask if blood clots are passed, and the quantity of tampons or sanitary towels which are required. Whilst some excessively fastidious women may change protection too often, it is a sure sign of menorrhagia when towels or tampons are used together or in pairs. If menorrhagia exists, an intrauterine device is unlikely to be a successful method for the woman and the condition itself may, in any case, require further investigation.

Health associated with the menstrual cycle
Before the onset of a period some women experience pre-menstrual tension. This may be expressed as a general state of irritability or labile emotional state, or may be more serious and result in severe depression or even violence. Migraine can also be a pre-menstrual problem. These conditions improve with certain forms of oral contraception and may be made worse by others.

Obstetric history

Details must be obtained about each pregnancy in order of occurrence with the length of gestation in each case. It is helpful to know if the pregnancies were planned; the health of the mother during pregnancy and subsequently; and the present health of each child. All pregnancies, regardless of outcome, should be included. Pregnancies resulting from contraceptive failure whatever their outcome, including termination, will require very careful enquiry into previous contraceptive practice.

Each pregnancy should be investigated for complications as a history of hypertension may predispose to a rise in blood pressure if oral contraception is decided upon. Thrombo–embolic disease should be noted because this is usually considered a contraindication for oral contraception.

The type of delivery should be noted: normal, forceps or caesarean section. A recent scar in the uterus requires consultant advice about the advisability of an IUD. A history of vaginal or pelvic floor trauma or a poorly healed episiotomy may be connected with dyspareunia.

When lactation is still occurring most doctors will avoid the use of combined oral contraceptives which may reduce the production of milk. The health of the children should be enquired into. If a child is mentally or physically handicapped or suffers an inherited disorder it may be necessary to widen the discussion to uncover particular anxieties about avoiding pregnancy, and sterilization could be indicated.

Gynaecological history

Details of any gynaecological condition are relevant to the choice of contraception. Enquiry should be made about past cervical smear results and surgery to the reproductive organs: vaginal repair, cervical amputation, cone biopsy, colposcopy, ectopic pregnancy and ovarian cysts should all be noted. A proven history of cancer is a contraindication to using combined oral contraception. These women should have consultant advice from the specialist responsible for their treatment. Whilst active pelvic inflammatory disease needs immediate investigation and treatment, chronic or quiescent disease may be activated by the insertion of an intrauterine device. Various failures to ovulate and the presence of ovarian cysts may be complicated by contraception, and fertility perhaps permanently affected. These women should seek advice from a gynaecologist. Recent history of hydatidiform mole will preclude oral contraception and IUD use until the results confirm that there is no recurrence of the disease.

Medical history

Jaundice and liver damage
It is important to note if any attack has occurred within the last six

to twelve months, and oral contraception is contraindicated whenever a serious attack is reported.

Thromboembolic disease
A history of this condition would usually be considered a complete contraindication for the use of a combined contraceptive pill. The progestogen-only pill may be a satisfactory alternative for women who particularly wish for oral contraception.

Cardiac conditions
Where the condition is requiring active treatment, specialist medical advice ought to be requested. Points of special concern are anticoagulants which would be affected by a combined pill, infection with a co-existing IUD leading to a septicaemia, and any method causing additional menstrual bleeding and predisposing to anaemia. However it is important to remember that considerable cardiac problems may result from an unplanned pregnancy.

Anaemia
This condition gives rise to general poor health and the cause should be investigated before proceeding. Some women with intrauterine devices lose more blood at menstruation, and some low-dose pills cause breakthrough bleeding which could theoretically worsen the position.

Drug therapy
Any regular drug therapy ought to be noted as interactions can occur with oral contraception and these are listed in section 7.2 (p. 61).

Carcinoma
Many forms of carcinoma, especially that occurring in the breast, respond adversely to oestrogen therapy and a specialist's advice should be obtained on the advisability of prescribing oral contraceptives.

Diabetes
Whilst there is no absolute contraindication, steroids contained in the contraceptive pill may upset insulin requirements and control so that diabetics are usually advised to consider alternative methods.

Thyroid deficiency

An underactive thyroid gland may cause scanty, irregular periods or menorrhagia, and contraception is best kept at the least hormonally invasive until the disease is diagnosed and treated.

Headaches and migraine

If these occur it is helpful to have details of their frequency and severity: they might not necessarily be a contraindication but may be thought to be side effects of oral contraception later on. They do, in fact, occasionally change their established pattern, for better or for worse.

Epilepsy

Unless fits are known to occur only during the pre-menstrual phase the condition is unlikely to be adversely affected by oral contraceptives. Drug interactions with epileptic-controlling drugs will need specialist opinion and control.

Allergies

These are not usually affected by oral contraception. Women with metal allergies may prefer to avoid copper bearing IUDs. Occasionally women may show a mild sensitivity to certain brands of spermicides.

Contact lens

The natural curvature of the cornea may alter slightly in a few cases where the pill causes mild fluid retention, and women should be warned that in a very few cases the lens may not fit as well as previously.

Hospital treatment as in- or out-patient

Enquiry about this may reveal important details not previously volunteered.

It would be as well to remember that the nurse herself comes under scrutiny and if she falls short of a woman's needs at an interview she will not be told the real problem. When a person is evidently unable to speak frankly about a problem, any questions which provoke stress such as the termination of a pregnancy or treatment of sexually transmitted diseases should not be asked too early in the interview: if unfortunately this happens and the response is not satisfactory, the nurse can repeat the question at the end of the interview when she feels she has gained the woman's confidence, in the hope of being given the true facts without cause for embarrassment. The nurse must listen carefully and with concern so that the woman is provided with the best opportunity of expressing herself freely. However, even with the most experienced staff, it is not unusual for some facts to escape only to find them given to someone else at a later date!

Family history

The occurrence of hypertension, diabetes, thromboembolic disease and breast cancer in the woman's immediate family should be noted and brought to the doctor's attention as this may put the client into a higher risk category for side effects if she chooses to try oral contraception.

To complete the history and confirm any anxieties that the woman may have expressed about being pregnant because of delayed menstruation a urine sample can be tested for pregnancy.

6.3 MEDICAL EXAMINATION

All women attending a clinic for the first time are carefully examined in order to detect the earliest sign of any condition which if overlooked could become a serious health hazard. Routine testing of weight and blood pressure are recorded, often before the formal examination.

Many doctors prefer to speak briefly to the woman before she undresses for the examination, as this establishes a more relaxed relationship. The doctor will need to be given all the woman's particulars and should have the opportunity to discuss any details with the nurse before examining the client. The nurse who has inter-viewed the woman should, where possible, remain with her for the examination. Every effort needs to be made to maintain dignity by ensuring privacy and adequate covering with some form of sheet.

In some clinics the examination is carried out entirely by the doctor; in others, the clinic nurse may be responsible for breast examination, vaginal inspection and cervical cytology, only draw-ing the doctor's attention to any abnormalities with which she may be concerned. The nurse will be shown how to perform these examinations during her practical training in family planning based on the following procedures.

Breast examination

Both breasts should be examined while the woman is sitting and again when she is lying on her back. The breasts should both be similar in size and any marked asymmetry or dimpling should be reported to the doctor. It is also important to notice the colour and texture of the skin and take serious note of patches of discoloration or leakage of fluid from the nipple. Each breast is then palpated for lumps, *using only the flat of the fingers*, and feeling in a circular direction from the nipple to the outer extremity, remembering to include the area under each axilla called the tail of spence (Figure 6.1).

During palpation the woman should lie flat on her back with the arm on the side being examined raised above her head on the pillow. When the examination is complete the nurse should enquire whether the woman does this examination herself, and if she wishes to be taught then the opportunity should be taken. It is best if self-examination is undertaken around the end of the first week of the cycle. Tissue growths, mostly benign but sometimes malignant, are common and women should consult their general practitioner without delay if they are worried about their own findings.

Genital inspection

In order to carry out this examination in the most relaxed manner it is important to ensure complete privacy. The client's external genitalia should be exposed only as much as is necessary for an adequate inspection and it is necessary to have a good directional source of light.

First the general appearance of the vulva is observed and any lesions or inflammation noted. Then an inspection of the vagina will enable the nurse to satisfy herself that it is healthy and normal. Details of how to pass a speculum and obtain a cervical smear are covered in sections 12.2 and 12.3.

6.4 CONCLUDING THE VISIT

When the examination and consultation with the doctor are complete and a satisfactory method of contraception has been

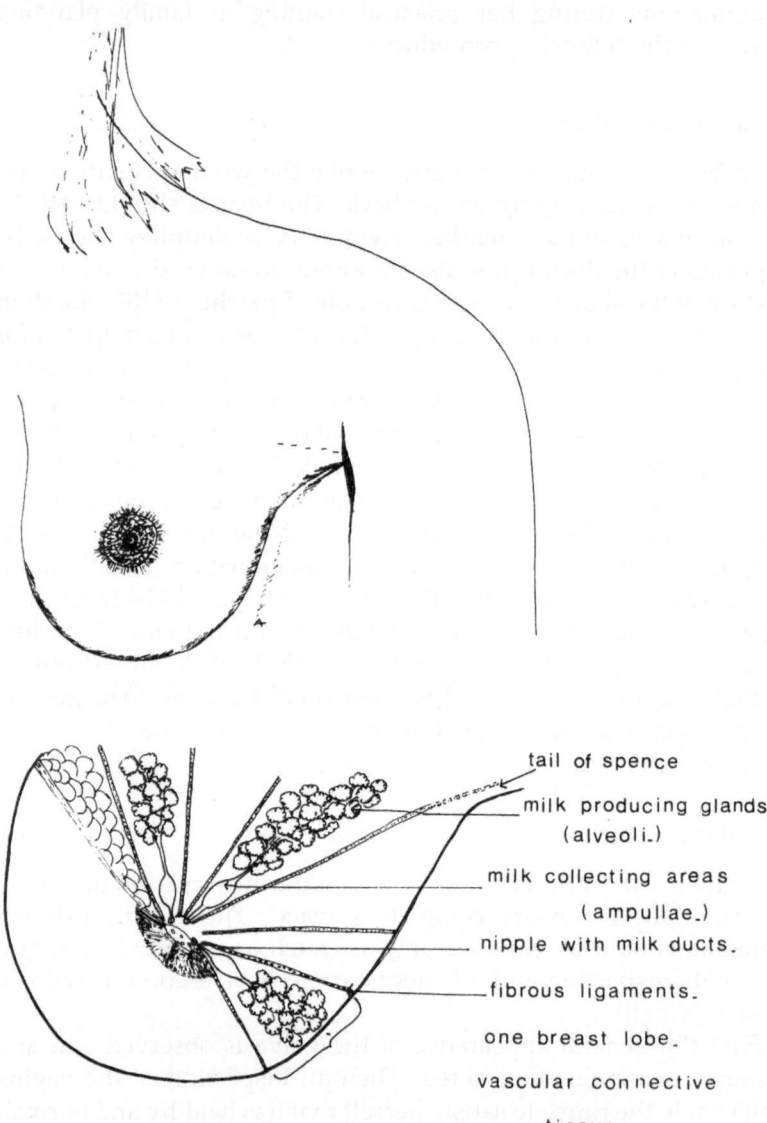

tail of spence

milk producing glands
(alveoli.)

milk collecting areas
(ampullae.)

nipple with milk ducts.

fibrous ligaments.

one breast lobe.

vascular connective
tissue.

Figure 6.1 Breast anatomy.

decided upon, it is the nurse's responsibility to make sure that the
woman understands the instructions for the safe use of the chosen

method. The possible side effects of the contraceptive method must be discussed and if she has not already collected a leaflet containing the appropriate information she should be given one to take away with her for reference purposes.

Details of the next appointment will be discussed with her and if she is given adequate reasons for returning it is likely that she will do so, and be contented with her chosen method of contraception. Other associated services available at the clinic should be outlined in case of future need.

7

Hormonal contraception

In the 25 years since the early 1960s oral contraception has proved itself to be an extremely efficient and generally accepted method of birth control. It is estimated that at present there are worldwide about 60 million women using this method.

The hormonal preparations used to prevent conception fall into two main groups, the first are those combining oestrogen and progestogen (the latter describes synthetic progesterone) and the second contain progestogen only. These alternatives will be described separately and details of some available preparations with their doses are given later in the chapter. Since their introduction there has been a gradual reduction in the quantity of both ingredients, including most recently the development of multi-phasic formulations which follow the pattern of the menstrual cycle as well as reducing the total intake of hormone each month.

7.1 TYPES OF ORAL CONTRACEPTIVE

1. Combined oestrogen and progestogen
   (a) *Monophasic*, consisting of 21 tablets of identical formula;
   (b) *Biphasic*, consisting of 21 tablets in two strengths;
   (c) *Triphasic*, consisting of 21 tablets in three strengths.
2. Progestogen only (mini-pill)
   (a) 28 tablets of equal strength;
   (b) 35 tablets of equal strength.
3. Post-coital
   2 × 2 tablets containing combined oestrogen and progestogen.

7.2 THE COMBINED PILL

The combined pill is the most widely used hormonal contraceptive in the United Kingdom today. When used correctly the risk of pregnancy is very low and estimated at 0.2/100 woman years. The strength of the pill was once described as high, medium or low dose according to the oestrogen content. Early preparations contained comparatively high doses of oestrogen (100 μg) but with time the quantities have been reduced and these original high-dose tablets are no longer available. The current maximum dose is, by comparison, a modest 50 μg of oestrogen, and many preparations range between 20 and 35 μg.

Numbers of drug companies have made efforts to produce an effective and safe pill with minimal side effects. This has resulted in a variety of strengths and combinations being available and marketed under different brand names. Consequently there are several preparations of almost identical dosage on the market, and some clinics and pharmacies have restricted the number of brands kept in stock. This may require explanation if a woman is given an identical preparation which has a different brand name from the one which she was previously receiving.

Table 7.1 Action of combined pill and progestogen-only pill

	Combined pill	Progestogen- only pill (POP)	Remarks
Inhibition of ovulation	+++	+ (in about 40% of cycles)	POP often causes amenorrhoea if ovulation is inhibited
Reduced sperm penetrability of cervical mucus	++	++	POP relies chiefly on this effect
Interference with tubal function (motility of tube, number and activity of cilia reduced)	++	+	Possible explanation for reported rise in ectopics with POP
Alteration of endometrial histology	+++	+	—
Contraceptive efficacy	++++ (approx. 0.2/100 WY)	++ (approx. 2/100 WY)	—

The action of the combined pill is to prevent the ovary from producing an ovum. This is achieved by oestrogen inhibiting the feedback mechanism to the hypothalamus which in turn prevents the anterior pituitary gland from producing follicle stimulating hormone (FSH). In addition the progestogen content of the pill causes cervical mucus, normally produced in quantity at the time of ovulation, to become dense and difficult for the sperm to penetrate. The quantity of oestrogen needed to suppress ovulation varies with individual women, and there is more positive control as the oestrogen content increases. The lowest dose pills keep such a delicate balance that it becomes vital for them to be taken at the same time each day.

Progestogen has few side effects and its benefits when taken as the progestogen-only pill (POP) are described later in this chapter (section 7.3). A summary of the action is given in Table 7.1.

Contraindications for the combined pill

When taking a full history on the woman's first visit to the clinic particular attention should be paid to contraindications, outlined here for guidance. It is obviously important to know of any existing conditions which would become worse with oestrogen therapy.

Absolute contraindications for the combined pill

> Oestrogen-dependent carcinoma
> Any history of thrombosis
> Recent liver disease

Risk factors with the combined pill

> Amenorrhoea (which may be due to pituitary dysfunction)
> Menstrual cycle only just established in young age group
> Severe migraine
> Epilepsy
> Diabetes
> Hypertension (diastolic pressure over 90 mm Hg)
> Hyperlipidaemia
> Heavy smoking habits
> Over 35 years of age
> Personal history of structural heart disease
> Family history of coronary heart disease/stroke

Obesity
Severe anxiety or depression
Anorexia nervosa
Lactation

Contraindicated before the situation is clarified

Irregular genital bleeding
Treated hydatidiform mole
Possible pregnancy
History of scanty menstrual loss and late menarche
Impending major surgery

Following the first visit, women are usually asked to return after their first three months on the pill to discuss any problems and satisfy themselves that all is well. Thereafter, regular attendances at the clinic should be arranged at six-monthly intervals; or more frequently if necessary. A record of blood pressure, weight and smoking habits should be made at all visits to the clinic.

The choice of a suitable pill is made by the doctor who, in the United Kingdom, is legally responsible for prescribing it. As already stated, the first prescription is usually given for a period of three months. When the woman returns to the clinic for a check-up after her first three months on the pill, the doctor, if he is satisfied with her condition, may prescribe a year's supply, at the same time stipulating the number of packets to be dispensed at that visit. Repeat packets of the prescribed pill can then be dispensed by the nurse at subsequent visits within the overall period covered by the prescription, provided of course that she is satisfied with the woman's general condition. On expiry of the full term of the prescription, the doctor must see the woman again before the prescription is renewed for a further period. Whilst the nurse cannot yet undertake the legal responsibility of prescribing or renewing oral contraceptives, she is responsible for monitoring the woman's progress, and therefore ought to, and often does, possess the knowledge to discuss intelligently alternative preparations which may be more suitable.

Teaching the use of the combined pill

Once the pill has been prescribed, the woman should be carefully instructed in its use. It is helpful to have some privacy to go through the details with her, and it greatly simplifies the task if a packet of the appropriate pills and an instruction sheet are to hand. The instruction sheet should be discussed and explained and a copy given to the woman to take home to read carefully and keep for reference.

There are two schools of thought about when the first course of pills is commenced. Both are given here, as methods A and B respectively. As doctors at different clinics vary in their choice of method, the nurse should ask the doctor with whom she is working which method he or she prefers and be flexible in teaching either of them.

Method A: commencing on day five
The first pill should be taken on the fifth day of the menstrual cycle, using an alternative method of contraception until the first seven pills have been taken (the manufacturer's recommendations may still state 14 days, but this is no longer considered essential). This is a useful method if the woman is menstruating at her first clinic visit.

Method B: commencing on day one
The first pill should be taken on the first day of the menstrual cycle; no alternative contraceptive method is needed. However, it is possible that the woman will experience some breakthrough bleeding with this method during the first cycle.

Each packet contains 21 pills with a seven-day break (with the exception of Mililyn which has 22 pills with a six day break, and Every Day (ED) preparations which include an additional seven inert tablets). It is important that the instructions are closely followed and that one pill is taken as regularly as possible at the same time each day, or within about six hours irrespective of the onset of any vaginal bleeding which will have been used as a previous monthly milestone, for after selecting the fifth day of the starting period there is no comparison in the timing of the cycles. It is most essential that the seven day interval is not inadvertently extended by forgetting the first or last pills. The woman should become familiar with the packet of pills she is to use and be allowed to examine it to see how the pills are wrapped and marked with the days of the week to enable her to check readily that she has taken the pill on the appropriate day.

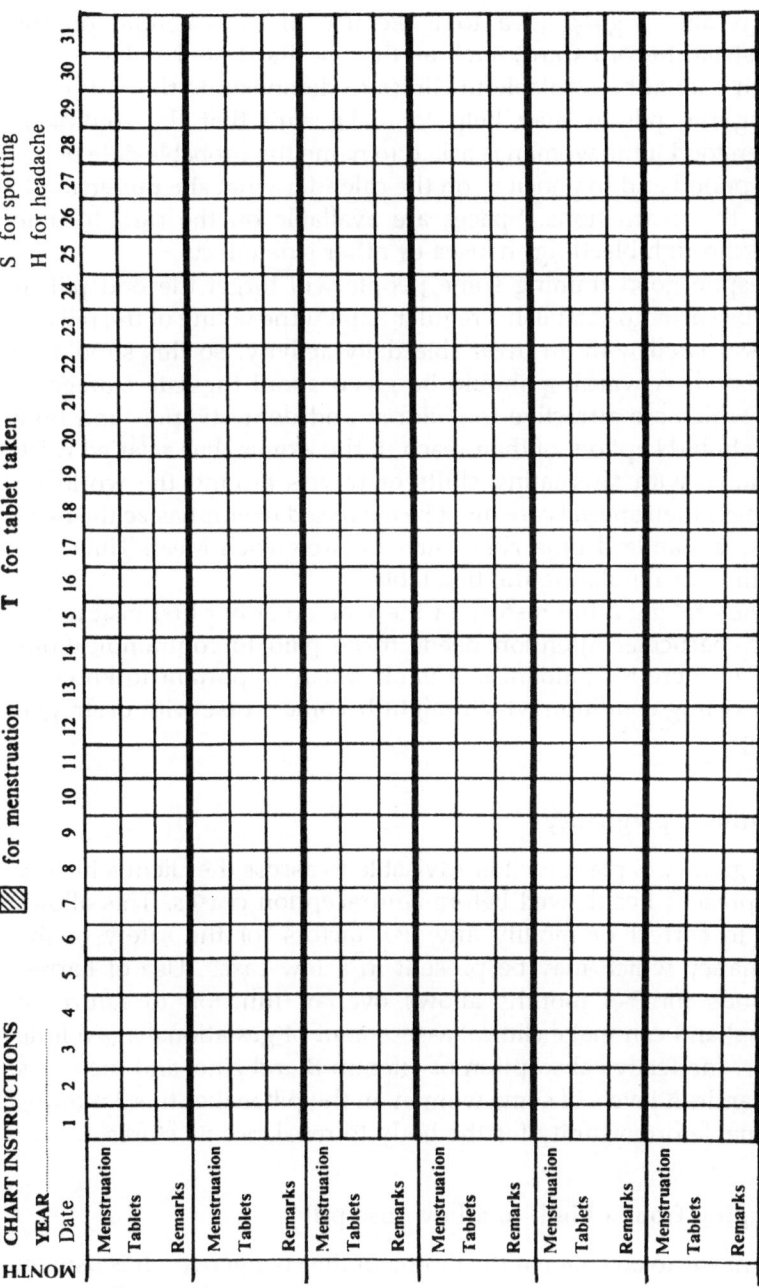

Figure 7.1 Menstrual record card.

It is also a good idea to make use of the calendar on the Menstrual Record Card, such as the one illustrated at Figure 7.1 which should be available in clinics to demonstrate the routine of taking the pill. It may help to make sure that the routine is understood if the woman is asked to name the probable date of her next period and to pencil in on the calendar what she understands from the instructions. Spaces are available on the card to note breakthrough bleeding, nausea or other side effects.

Despite good training some people will forget the odd pill. It may be easier to establish a regular habit if the taking of the pill can be associated with an invariable daily activity, so this should be discussed. A warning should be given about the safe storage of pills which are attractive to children and domestic pets and how they should kept out of their reach. If the woman has a varied work timetable with alternating shifts or travels around the world on business then special care must be exercised to emphasize the need to use a standard time zone such as Greenwich Mean Time as a baseline for regulating the timetable.

When taking a full history of the woman at her first visit to the clinic, particular attention needs to be paid to contraindications outlined here for guidance. It is obviously important to know of any existing condition which might become worse with oestrogen therapy.

Planning a pregnancy

If pregnancy is planned it is advisable to assess the client's history and present health well before contraception ceases. This allows time to correct or modify any risk factors for the safety of the pregnancy which may be present in a few cases. Use of barrier methods for 3–6 months allows ovarian function to return to normal and can make clinical assessment of gestational age a little easier. Ineffective absorption of vitamin B and zinc, and increases in vitamin A levels of some women on the pill makes this 3 months a valuable opportunity for the body to rebalance its stores.

Changing from a high- to a low-dose pill

Care needs to be taken in the timing of the changeover. It is usually best for the currently used packet of higher dose pills to be completed before a new packet of low-dose pills is commenced, and the change should take place without a break. The new packet of low-dose pills should be continued for 21 days followed by a 7 day break, and then the routine of taking 21 pills followed by a 7 day break should be continued. If the woman is changing to an ED version then the inactive tablets should be disregarded and the new preparation should be commenced with the appropriate day's active tablet taken from the red sector of the pack and continued in sequence without interruption.

In the case of changing to a progestogen-only pill, the 7 day break should likewise be omitted and the new packet started immediately after the combined oral contraceptive pill cycle is completed.

There may or may not be breakthrough bleeding during the switchover. Either way, the woman can rest assured that she is safe from pregnancy if she has followed the instructions closely. However, a warning should be included that it is possible for pregnancy to occur during the changeover if the instructions are not followed carefully.

The forgotten pill

If one pill is forgotten it should be taken as soon as possible. If more than 12 hours have elapsed then one should be taken at once and the regime continued but with extra contraceptive precautions being taken for at least seven days. If several pills have been omitted then medical advice should be sought. It is usually advisable to start a new packet at once and omit the interval between the current course and the next packet. Irregular vaginal bleeding is likely to result from erratic use of the pill. This may take time to settle down and very occasionally the prescription has to be discontinued for a short time whilst the endometrial cycle recovers.

The missed pills which are most likely to result in an unplanned pregnancy are those at the beginning and end of the packet, because extending the seven pill-free days allows the pituitary to release FSH which subsequently can cause a breakthrough ovulation. When pills are forgotten towards or at the end of a course the next packet should be taken in continuity without the usual seven day break. A more difficult situation exists when the first few pills are accidentally omitted. The advice extends to the immediate use of barrier methods for a minimum of seven days by which time the level of protection will have risen to the comparative safety of the POP and this will be sustained until the next expected cyclical vaginal bleeding.

There are three alternatives for the forgetful woman. The simplest is to prescribe an Every Day (ED) preparation which has an extra seven inert tablets, one for each day of the usual break; unfortunately only a limited number of preparations are produced with this facility. The second approach to this problem is to reduce the usual seven day break between packets to five days which maintains cycle control. The final alternative is to use a preparation containing 50 μg of oestrogen which has a more assertive influence.

Occasionally, problems may arise if there is a delay in collecting the next prescription, but possession of a reserve packet will usually prevent the risky practice of borrowing from friends. Breakthrough bleeding is quite common when pills are taken irregularly. This may be slight but is likely to last for up to five or six days, and in spite of this the pill must be continued.

Menstrual blood loss

After oral contraception is commenced the periods usually become much lighter because the endometrium remains in a primitive condition and there is less tissue to shed. The blood loss is due to hormone withdrawal and this may tend to reduce the quantity lost until it becomes scanty. A few women cease to lose blood altogether and should be advised that if this happens two months in succession they should seek advice from their doctor. However, unless pills have been omitted or other drug therapy has interfered with the hormone regime, pregnancy is unlikely. Women using hormonal contraception seem to benefit from a marked reduction in pre-menstrual tension and absence of dysmenorrhoea.

Drug interactions

One drug may influence the absorption of another in several ways, and this is especially the case when low-dose pills are in use. Several common drugs such as antibiotics and barbiturates reduce the efficacy of the contraceptive pill and make the user vulnerable to pregnancy. If a course of antibiotics is prescribed the pill should be continued, but other precautions should also be taken and continued until the antibiotic treatment is completed and at least seven more pills have been taken. This does not apply to all

Table 7.2 Drug interactions with oral contraception

Analgesics and anti-inflammatory agents

Pyrazole group
Amidopyrine (aminophenazone)
Oxyphenbutazone
Phenazone (antipyrene)
Phenylbutazone

Possible reduction of
  contraceptive efficacy

Ethylmorphine

Possible reduction of
  contraceptive efficacy

Pethidine (meperidine)

Possible increase of
  sensitivity to pethidine,
  i.e. increased analgesia and
  CNS depression

Phenacetin

Possible reduction of
  contraceptive efficacy

Anginal drugs and coronary vasodilators
Clofibrate

Theoretically possible that
  contraceptive efficacy
  could be reduced

Anticoagulants
Anticoagulants

Possible reduction in the
  effect of anticoagulants and
  dosage of these may need
  to be increased

Anticonvulsants

Hydantoins
Ethotoin
Methoin
Phenytoin (diphenylhydantoin)

Ethosuximide

Primidone

Possible reduction of
  contraceptive efficacy
  (patients with epilepsy
  should be observed
  carefully during oral
  contraceptive use for
  signs of fluid retention)

Antidepressants

Tricyclics
Imipramine

Decrease in therapeutic effect
  of imipramine and increase
  in toxic response, such as
  mammary hypertrophy
  any galactorrhoea

(continued)

Table 7.2 *continued*

Antihistamines
Chlorcyclizine   Possible reduction of
                                        contraceptive efficacy

Antihypertensives
Cyclopenthiazide   Possible reduction of anti-
                                        hypertensive efficacy
Guanethidine   (contraceptive-induced
                                        hypertension may be
                                        refactory to guanethidine)

Methyldopa   Possible reduction of anti-
                                        hypertension efficacy and
                                        possible potentiation of
                                        mammotropic side-effects
                                        of methyldopa

Reserpine   Possible potentiation of
                                        mammotropic side-effects
                                        of reserpine

Anti-infective agents
Ampicillin
Chloramphenicol
Neomycin
Nitrofurantoin
Penicillin V (phenoxymethyl   Possible reduction of
  penicillin)   contraceptive efficacy
Rifampicin
Sulphamethoxypyridazine

Barbiturates
Hexobarbitone   Possible reduction of
Phenobarbitone   contraceptive efficacy
Methylphenobarbitone   (especially
                                        methylphenobarbitone)

Corticosteroids
Corticosteroids (systemic)   Dosage adjustment
                                        (reduction) of
                                        corticosteroids may
                                        be necessary

Table 7.2 *continued*

Gastrointestinal sedatives	
Hyoscine	Possible reduction of contraceptive efficacy
Haemostatic agents	
Aminocaproic acid	Possible development of hypercoagulable state
Hypnotics (see also barbiturates)	
Chloral hydrate and its derivatives	
Chloral glycerolate	Theoretically these known
Dichloralphenazone	enzyme-inducers could
Ethchlorvynol	increase rate of oestrogen
Methaqualone	metabolism and possibly reduce efficacy of oral contraceptive
Hypoglycaemic agents	
Insulin	Patients should be carefully
Oral hypoglycaemic agents	observed as control of diabetes may be reduced
Muscle relaxants	
Orphenadrine	Possible reduction of contraceptive efficacy
Sedatives and tranquillizers	
Chlorpromazine	Possible reduction of
Meprobamate	contraceptive efficacy
Chlorprothixene	Possible potentiation of mammotropic side-effects of chlorprothixene
Chlordiazepoxide	Possible reduction of contraceptive efficacy and possible potentiation of mammotropic side-effects of chlordiazepoxide
Vasoconstrictors and migraine treatments	
Dihydroergotamine	Possible reduction of contraceptive efficacy

(continued)

Table 7.2 *continued*

Ergotamine	Rare possibility of predisposing to the development of deep vein thrombosis. (Patients with migraine should be observed carefully during oral contraception use for signs of fluid retention.)

antibiotics but women should be advised to seek the doctor's advice at the time he prescribes. A list of drug interactions is provided in Table 7.2.

Antibiotics alter the normal bacterial flora in the intestine and a more rapid passage of the bowel contents tends to impair the ability of the body to absorb hormones through the gut wall. Some drugs, including barbiturates, enhance liver enzyme activity and the hormones are therefore more rapidly broken down and excreted. In some cases the hormones may block the excretion of the other drug in the liver and increase its concentration in the body beyond a level which is safe or desirable. Alternatively, the presence of hormones may reduce the effect of the drug and a larger dose may be necessary. Impaired drug absorption and function can be indicated by breakthrough bleeding where the pills have been taken regularly. If the woman mentions this problem she should be asked about other medication and a doctor's advice sought. All episodes of breakthrough bleeding, unless associated with the forgotten pill, should be considered as an indication that the dosage of the pill is insufficient and a higher dose is probably required.

The efficacy of the contraceptive pill will also be reduced if there is a gastrointestinal infection or disturbance. If a pill is vomited another should be taken as soon as possible, and if diarrhoea occurs then it must be considered that the hormones may not have been properly absorbed and additional contraceptive measures will be necessary. Women planning holidays abroad may be wise to consider the increased risk of gastric upsets resulting from the change of diet, e.g. over-indulgence of rich and unfamiliar foods or impure water. Gastrointestinal disturbance on holiday is distressing; being unable to procure any male or female barrier methods of contraception as an extra precaution may be disastrous. A gentle reminder to take a cap and spermicide or a few condoms may be the saving of the holiday.

Side effects

A summary of side effects and recommended treatment is given in Table 7.3.

Table 7.3 Management of oral contraceptive side-effects

Side effect	Suggested action	
	Oestrogen	Progestogen
Acne	reduce	
Amenorrhoea (not pregnant)		increase
Bloating	reduce	
Breakthrough bleeding		increase
Breast discomfort	reduce	reduce
Depression		reduce
Headache (not migraine)		increase
Heavy bleeding		increase
Hypertension	reduce	
Loss of libido		reduce
Migraine (recurrent)		reduce
Nausea	reduce	
Pre-menstrual tension		reduce
Weight gain	reduce	reduce

Hypertension
A rise in blood pressure may become evident within a few months of commencing the combined pill. In most cases the onset is gradual and if the contraceptive is changed – for instance, from a high to a low-dose pill – this is sometimes effective in reducing the blood pressure back to normal. Women over 35 years of age and women of any age who smoke are more likely to have hyper-tension. The blood pressure of all women on the combined pill should be monitored every six months, or more frequently if there is any rise causing concern. Some women become very anxious before a clinic visit and this can affect the systolic reading. After the woman has been seen the blood pressure may be checked either at

the clinic or by her own doctor on another occasion in an environment where she is more relaxed.

Thromboembolic incidence

The publicity which thromboembolism has received makes this a very common anxiety amongst women. In fact, it is quite rare and not always due to the pill. The effect of oestrogen may cause the blood platelets to become a little stickier than normal, just as they do in pregnancy, and therefore there is a predisposition to clot. When this is coupled with venous stasis caused by varicose veins or prolonged bed-rest, especially associated with surgery, the risk is greatly increased. The combined pill is not prescribed for women who give a past history of thromboembolism because of the increased risk. However, it must be remembered that any unplanned pregnancy could produce a similar risk of clotting.

Weight gain

Some weight gain may be noticed initially. This is due to an alteration in body metabolism and can usually be effectively controlled by reducing carbohydrate and starchy foods in the daily diet. A slight increase in body fluids may also occur as the body adjusts itself. The lower the hormone level the less likelihood there is of a gain in weight.

Headaches

A few people find that they suffer from headaches, but these may not be directly associated with oral contraception. In some cases, however, they are thought to be due to progestogen withdrawal, often noticed during the pill-free week, and the condition is relieved if the pill is taken continuously or if extra progestogen is taken between cycles. Persistent complaints of severe headache must be properly investigated.

Nausea

A few women may complain of nausea but this rarely lasts more than the first month. It may be possible to influence the effect by changing the time that the pill is taken.

Chloasma

If this occurs it is generally slight. The pigmentation change appearing on the face is also seen in pregnancy, and resembles a patchy sunburn on the forehead and cheeks. In very sunny environments the use of a wide-brimmed hat and shading will minimize the effect in those persons who are susceptible. A good filtering sunscreen cream can also be used. Unlike the chloasma which clears after pregnancy, it does not disappear when the pill is discontinued: it fades gradually and may take months or even years to clear.

Acne
The low-dose pills containing norgestrel can aggravate acne but Minovlar and Minilyn improve it. Dyane is specifically marketed for skin conditions and has a useful contraceptive effect.

Vaginal discharge
Candida albicans or thrush may be encouraged and difficult to treat because the acidity of the vagina is reduced by the combined pill just as it is in pregnancy. In extreme cases it may be necessary to find an alternative method of contraception. Some women are concerned about excessive vaginal secretions which are sometimes a nuisance; however a little reassurance is all that is required.

Depression
Some women experience depression when taking the pill. Pyridoxine (vitamin B_6) may be useful but the doctor may decide that the depression is due to external factors. If antidepressants need to be prescribed, alternative contraception should be commenced.

Stress
A woman who has been persuaded to use oral contraception by her family, friends or medical adviser and who is not really happy about it will come to the clinic with a variety of problems, some of which are a direct result of the stress and anxiety felt in taking something about which she is uncertain. Special care should be taken to understand her doubts and misgivings and she will require help to accept and appreciate the benefits of contraception. The media is sometimes responsible for causing public concern and stress to women using contraceptives, and in order to be prepared for this anyone working in the field is advised to keep in touch with this source of information. From time to time the waves of public anxiety are aroused by a newspaper article or television programme which immediately brings a burst of enquiries to the

clinics. These enquiries need to be met with sympathetic and informed advice, and careful explanation and reassurance should be offered. In some cases it may be more helpful to try another method.

In general most women who are really well motivated and confident about oral contraception remain remarkably well and happy and experience few side effects.

7.3 THE PROGESTOGEN-ONLY PILL (POP)

The second group of hormonal preparations contains synthetic progesterone in the form of progestogen. The progestogen-only pill has the advantage of eliminating altogether the side effects of oestrogen experienced with the combined pill, whilst maintaining a very high effectiveness. The risk of a pregnancy at 2–3/100 woman years is only marginally higher than that of the combined pill and compares favourably with the IUD. It is a reliable and satisfactory method for women who are not tolerating the combined pill very well, or who are developing hypertension. It is a particularly good method for women over 35 years of age who have been on the combined pill and are concerned about the increased risk of circulatory disease. As they become older the risk increases with a corresponding reduction in fertility which makes the POP a very acceptable alternative contraceptive. The method is good for recently delivered mothers as unlike the combined counterpart it does not diminish lactation and is especially useful at this vulnerable time for the mother and her family. Diabetic patients may also find that their condition is easier to control using the single progestogen rather than the oestrogen-containing combined pill.

The action of progestogen is threefold:

1. It causes changes in the cervical mucus which becomes thick and sticky with entangled molecular structure and this forms a plug in the cervical canal which is an effective barrier against the sperm gaining access to the uterine cavity.
2. The drug also causes the endometrium to become atrophied and this reduces its ability to nourish an ovum should it become fertilized and attempt to embed itself in the uterus.
3. It affects the motility of the fallopian tube so that the transport of the ovum in the tube is slower. This may also help to prevent

conception; it could, however, contribute to the risk of ectopic pregnancy.

Sometimes the progestogen disturbs the normal ovulatory pattern and causes some cycles to be anovular, but this is only intermittent. The cycles are, however, irregular both in spacing and in quantity of menstrual products and so some women may find it difficult to adjust. A woman who already has a history of irregular or scanty menstrual cycles, or who has been investigated for infertility associated with abnormal ovulatory function may not be a suitable candidate for the POP.

Teaching the use of progestogen-only pill

The pill is commenced on the first day of the menstrual cycle and should be taken regularly at the same hour each day; preferably in the early evening, as it is at maximum concentration in body tissues about four hours afterwards. It should be continued without any break for as long as contraception is desired. Additional contraceptive precautions should be used for the first 48 hours of the first packet of pills. It is essential to go on taking the pills even when menstruation is occurring in order to maintain the effective level. Some women find daily pills without a break easier to remember and are more reliable about taking them regularly.

A certain number of women on the progestogen pill will become aware of a change in the pattern of their periods, which tend to become irregular. In addition they may experience irregular and quite frequent episodes of breakthrough bleeding, which indicates that they are probably ovulating although some cycles are anovular. As they continue with the pills the periods will become scanty and may eventually become almost non-existent. In a few cases the periods may cease altogether. This can alarm some women and it may be helpful if the full physiology is explained in advance so they are clear about how progestogens function. Women will be reassured to know that amenorrhoea is an indication of suppression of ovulation. In spite of this reassurance it may be as well, at a subsequent visit, to teach the women who need it how to distinguish the early signs of pregnancy, such as frequency of micturition, breast enlargement and tenderness, nausea and weight gain combined with amenorrhoea. This will help to avoid unnecessary anxiety if amenorrhoea should develop.

It also reminds the clinic staff of the signs and symptoms about which particular attention should be paid in case of genuine method failure. If a woman is still seriously concerned and has not had a period for eight weeks she should contact her own doctor or come to the clinic for a medical examination, bringing with her a specimen of urine passed first thing in the morning for pregnancy testing. It should be borne in mind that ordinary pregnancy tests on urine are unreliable until at least ten days after the expected period which has been missed.

When she decides to stop the POP, the woman should be advised, if she is menstruating, to continue taking the tablets until the next period.

Whilst it is rare to have to change from a POP to a combined oral contraceptive it is recommended that the changeover is carried out without a break on the first day of any menstruation. In those cases where menstruation has not been occurring for some months the direct change from one packet to the other can take place at any convenient time.

The forgotten pill

If a pill is forgotten, it should be taken as soon as possible, even if two have to be taken in the one day. The safety of the method is obviously reduced if pills are forgotten; so if more than three hours have elapsed extra precautions with sheaths and pessaries should also be used for two days during which two more pills will have been properly taken.

7.4 POST-COITAL CONTRACEPTION

Post-coital contraception is better known as 'the morning after pill'. Where unprotected intercourse has taken place it is possible to provide a fair amount of protection by offering a large dose of oestrogen as soon after the event as possible, and in any case within 72 hours. Two tablets of a preparation containing levonorgestrel 250 μg with ethinyl-oestradiol 50 μg are taken, and repeated after twelve hours. Before prescribing it is essential to make sure that there are no contraindications to oestrogen therapy, and the woman ought to be advised that she may feel slightly nauseated. It is important to offer the warning that if menstruation has not happened inside three weeks further medical assessment and advice must be sought.

Suitable preparations include tablets taken from a course of Eugynon 50 or Ovran and PC4 which is a purpose packaged preparation containing four tablets and full instructions.

In some cases a doctor may insert an intrauterine device within five days of unprotected intercourse as a post-coital method of avoiding pregnancy if fertilization has occurred. It is certainly prudent to arrange a pregnancy test whenever there is doubt. Recently it has become possible to have a positive result as early as one week after the period was due, but a negative result should be confirmed a week to ten days later.

Research has shown a 97.5% success rate in the use of post-coital contraception. However, there is a positive correlation between failure rate and the number of previous pregnancies when the oral contraceptive method is used.

7.5 INTRAMUSCULAR PREPARATIONS

Women who benefit from this method are those who require a highly efficient short term contraceptive. It is a particularly good method of preventing an unplanned pregnancy in the three months following rubella immunization, when there are high chances of risking fetal abnormality. Another use is in those women who plan to be sterilized because their usual method is no longer acceptable or safe and who are grateful to be provided with protection whilst the operation is arranged. Some women require a short term protection whilst their husbands wait for their sterilization to be pronounced effective as there is a delay between vasectomy and absence of any sperm in the ejaculate. Occasionally it may be the only acceptable method and can be used for long periods by domiciliary family planning staff. The relief it provides in having better spacing between children greatly reduces the mortality and morbidity risks for the mother and her children.

The commonest preparation is Depot Provera (medroxy-progesterone acetate) which is usually given in a dose of 150 mg every 3 months or 90 days. The other preparation, Norigest (norethisterone oenanthate), is given every eight weeks in doses of 200 mg. Both preparations are first injected during menstruation to avoid effects on an unknown pregnancy and the high level of progestogen suppresses ovulation in the same way as the combined pill. The method is very safe with the advantages of a pregnancy rate less than 1 per 100 woman years and few side effects. The main disadvantage is amenorrhoea which sometimes

Table 7.4 Oestrogen and progestogen preparations

Pill type	Preparation	Manufacturer	Oestrogen (µg)	Progestogen (mg)	
Combined					
Ethinyloestradiol/ norethisterone type	Loestrin 20	Parke-Davis	20	1	norethisterone acetate*
	Loestrin 30	Parke-Davis	30	1.5	norethisterone acetate*
	Conova 30	Gold Cross	30	2	ethynodiol diacetate*
	Brevinor	Syntex	35	0.5	norethisterone
	Ovysmen	Ortho-Cilag	35	0.5	norethisterone
	Neocon 1/35	Ortho-Cilag	35	1	norethisterone
	Norimin	Syntex	35	1	norethisterone
	Minovlar (also ED)	Schering	50	1	norethisterone acetate
	Minilyn	Organon	50	2.5	lynoestrenol*
	Gynovlar 21	Schering	50	3	norethisterone acetate
Ethinyloestradiol/ levonorgestrel	Microgynon 30	Schering	30	0.15	
	Ovranette	Wyeth	30	0.15	
	Eugynon 30	Schering	30	0.25	
	Ovran 30	Wyeth	30	0.25	
	Eugynon 50	Schering	50	0.5	norgestrel
	Ovran	Wyeth	50	0.25	
Ethinyloestradiol/ desogestrel	Marvelon	Organon	30	0.15	
	Mercilon	Organon	20	0.15	
Ethinyloestradiol/ gestodene	Femodene	Schering	30	0.075	
	Minulet	Wyeth	30	0.075	
Mestranol/ norethisterone	Norinyl-1	Syntex	50	1	
	Ortho-Novin 1/50	Ortho-Cilag	50	1	

Pill type	Preparation	Manufacturer	Oestrogen (μg)	Progestogen (mg)	
Biphasic and Triphasic					
Ethinyloestradiol/ norethisterone	Binovum	Ortho-Cilag	35	0.5	(7 tabs)
			35	1	(14 tabs)
	Synphase	Syntex	35	0.5	(7 tabs)
			35	1	(9 tabs)
			35	0.5	(5 tabs)
	Trinovum	Ortho-Cilag	35	0.5	(7 tabs)
			35	0.75	(7 tabs)
			35	1	(7 tabs)
Ethinyloestradiol/ levonorgestrel	Logynon (also ED)	Shering	30	0.05	(6 tabs)
			40	0.075	(5 tabs)
			30	0.125	(10 tabs)
	Trinordiol	Wyeth	30	0.05	(6 tabs)
			40	0.075	(5 tabs)
			30	0.125	(10 tabs)
Progestogen only					
Norethisterone type	Micronor	Ortho-Cilag	–	0.35	norethisterone
	Noriday	Syntex	–	0.35	norethisterone
	Femulen	Gold Cross	–	0.5	ethynodiol diacetate*
Levonorgestrel	Microval	Wyeth	–	0.03	
	Norgeston	Schering	–	0.03	
	Neogest	Schering	–	0.075	norgestrel

*Converted (>90%) to norethisterone as the active metabolite.

occurs after two injections. Any delay in recommencing ovulation is more pronounced following the use of Depot Provera than Norigest. Caution should be observed in offering this contraception in the postpartum period because the occasional bleeding episodes which can occur are more likely to do so in the first 6 weeks after delivery, and would confuse the diagnostic picture.

7.6 SUMMARY

Despite waves of concern when various research results are reported in the media, systemic contraception has a good safety record and is an extremely popular method of birth control. Details of various commercially available preparations are given in Table 7.4.

8

Barriers and spermicides

Barrier methods of contraception, as the name implies, are those which provide a mechanical barrier between the sperm and the ovum. This form of contraception has a long history and details of very bizarre and amusing objects which have been used for this purpose can be found dating far back into the past and make colourful reading. The fact that barrier methods are still in use today shows their importance and viability. When used correctly in conjunction with spermicide, which adds a chemical barrier, they are satisfactory and produce very few side effects. They do however depend on good motivation for successful use.

8.1 MALE BARRIER METHODS

Sheaths to cover the erect penis were originally made from leather and animal gut; they were washed and used many times. Now manufactured in latex, they are disposable after a single use and are probably the commonest method of contraception in the UK. Their popularity (Figure 8.1) is partly due to the ease with which they can be obtained from barbers, chemists, supermarkets, slot machines and from family planning clinics. Where men prefer to have the control over contraception they can do so privately, without the need to seek medical advice. Another advantage of the sheath over other alternative methods of contraception is that it provides some protection from sexually transmitted diseases. The sheaths are known by a variety of other names – condoms, rubbers, french letters and Durex (which is a trade name). Sheaths are made of plain latex in a variety of thicknesses and shapes and are now disposable and should only be used once. During manufacture they are electronically tested to ensure that not even

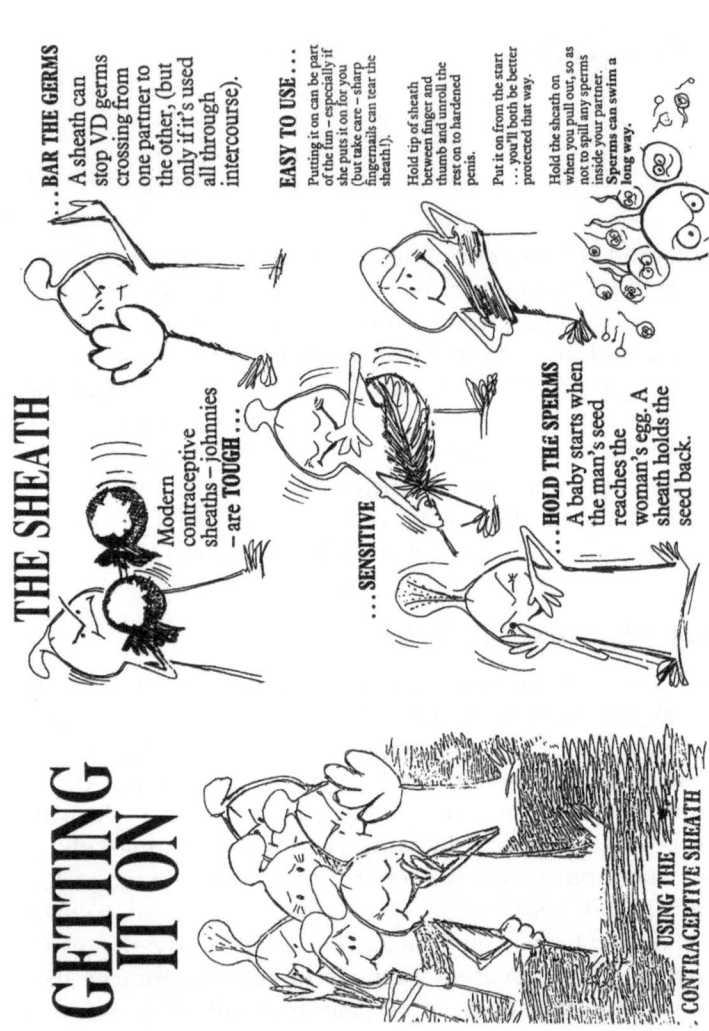

Figure 8.1 The sheath.

the smallest hole passes the high standard of quality control. The majority of sheaths are smooth, but some are ridged, being designed to help couples who complain of reduced sensation. Some sheaths are round–ended whilst others end in a small teat. The teat is designed to catch the ejaculate, and should be compressed between finger and thumb to exclude air when the sheath is being applied to the erect penis. The round–ended ones should also be compressed for about 1 cm at the tip as the space gives room for the ejaculated fluid and sperm and reduces the risk of splitting. Sheaths may also be purchased in many different colours. The rainbow packets create fun and are popular with couples of all ages and have been known to bring a twinkle into the eye of the most erudite professor! With improved methods of manufacture most sheaths are now prelubricated, and a recent innovation has been the production of a sheath which has the lubricant impregnated with spermicide. Those people allergic to rubber may obtain sheaths with a non-allergic finish on request at chemists.

The use of the sheath

As previously mentioned, sheaths are electronically tested when manufactured and, in the United Kingdom, stringent controls are maintained by the appropriate BSI (British Standards Institute) licence. The sheaths are very fine and can be damaged quite easily if not handled correctly. They are individually packed, rolled up and ready to use. Rough hands or sharp finger nails can easily tear the delicate latex, so it is essential to be gentle when removing them from the wrapper.

The sheath should be applied to the erect penis before any genital contact has taken place between the couple. The teat, or end, is compressed to remove air, and the sheath carefully rolled back over the full length of the shaft of the penis. It should remain covering the penis during intercourse and afterwards the sheath should be held in place on withdrawing the now flaccid penis from the vagina so that no ejaculate is spilt on or near the vulva. Only one sperm is necessary to fertilize an ovum whilst several hundred million are passed in each ejaculation and so care is essential. It is helpful if both partners understand the method correctly and women are recommended to insert a spermicide at a convenient time a little before intercourse. Manufacturers do not recommend the use of all spermicides as a few have been known to damage the latex. It is advisable to remind people to use only the spermicides provided by the clinic and if necessary obtain the same brands from their chemists. Petroleum jelly must be avoided.

Many couples use the sheath regularly as their own choice. It has also proved to be an excellent short term contraceptive method providing an additional precaution while the woman is changing from one type of contraceptive to another.

8.2 FEMALE BARRIER METHODS

A variety of caps and diaphragms have been designed for women (Figure 8.2). Each type covers the cervix and provides a barrier against sperm. They are popular with couples who have a regular pattern of intercourse, but are less easy to use when the pattern is unpredictable or where there is little privacy.

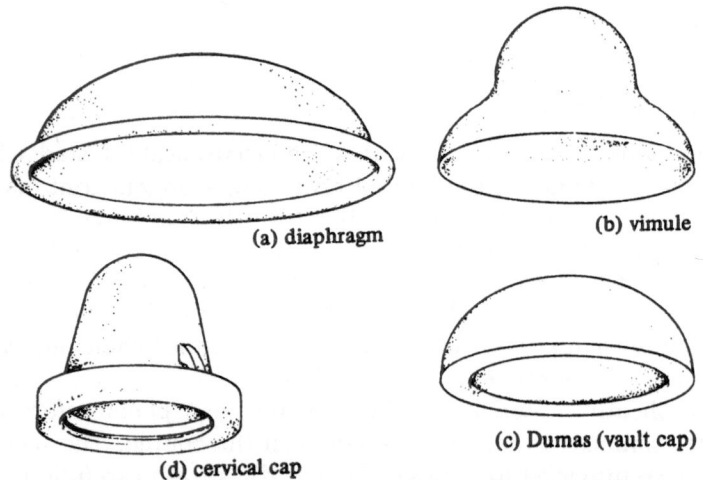

(a) diaphragm

(b) vimule

(c) Dumas (vault cap)

(d) cervical cap

Figure 8.2 Examples of female barrier methods.

The diaphragm or Dutch cap

This is the most commonly used female barrier method. It is made of thin latex which is dome-shaped and supported on a circular metal spring. Caps are graduated in size from 50 mm increasing in 5 mm steps up to 95 mm. An average size is 75 mm. The smallest and largest sizes are seldom used. The size of the cap needed varies for each individual and requires careful vaginal examination to assess the length from the posterior fornix of the vagina to behind the pubic bone. The doctor or nurse making this assessment selects the most likely size and inserts it so that it fits across the cervix, resting posteriorly in the fornix and anteriorly on the ledge behind the pubic bone (Figure 8.3). If properly fitted the woman will be unaware of its presence and it will not be felt by the partner during intercourse.

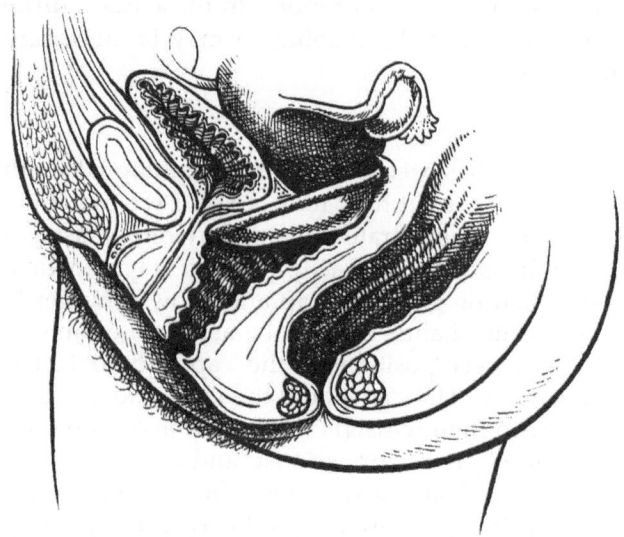

Figure 8.3 Diaphragm cap in position.

The initial cap fitting always needs checking in a week's time and again in two to three months. Some women are very tense, and the presence of vaginissmus (painful spasm of the vagina) may result in too small a diaphragm being fitted. This can be changed for a larger size when the woman returns to the clinic the following week in a more relaxed condition. In order to provide complete protection, the diaphragm must be a firm fit and be inserted correctly. If the size is too small it will move around so that the man's penis can accidentally enter above the cap, or cap itself may rest between the cervix and the pubic bone and fail to cover the cervix. If too large, it will not remain behind the pubic bone and will cause discomfort for both partners whilst affording no protection from pregnancy. Poor vaginal muscle tone or a shallow pubic ridge may make accurate fitting difficult: occasionally the flat spring becomes distorted and the imperfect fit will give poor protection. In these cases a coiled spring may fit more snugly. Arcing spring caps are also useful and are much easier for the woman to insert.

The most careful reassessment of all will be needed for women who remain tense at the first follow-up visit, for post-natal women and for those who have been dieting and losing weight or who have gained seven pounds or more. In these cases further checks on the size and fit of the diaphragm may be necessary at more frequent intervals.

Teaching the use of the diaphragm
The woman who has been fitted with a diaphragm by either doctor or nurse must be taught how to insert and remove it herself. It is often helpful to demonstrate the anatomy on a plastic model and show her with a small cap exactly where it is lying when inserted. She should then be given the cap and shown the flexibility of it. After washing her hands she can be asked to examine herself to identify the correct position of the cap and to feel the cervix through the dome. The cap should then be removed, preferably by the woman who then reinserts it. The cap is compressed between finger and thumb, dome uppermost, and inserted backwards and downwards in a similar way to inserting a tampon. The posture adopted in order to insert it may be varied; squatting is often easiest, but some people prefer to stand with one leg raised on a stool. When the cap has been inserted the woman is asked to examine herself to see if the cap is correctly positioned and covering the cervix. After this insertion has been checked by the nurse the cap is removed.

The handling of the cap is an acquired skill because of the spring in the rim, and as the application of spermicide tends to make it slippery this should be omitted until the necessary dexterity has been developed. Therefore during this learning period of about one week the method must not be relied upon. The woman is encouraged to practise daily at home and if the cap is difficult to insert dry it may be moistened under the tap or with a very little KY jelly applied to the leading edge.

When she is sure that the diaphragm can be inserted and

removed correctly the nurse should instruct the woman in cleaning and storing the diaphragm. It should be rinsed in warm water and dried carefully, inspected for damage and adjusted to a circular shape before being placed in its box. If powder is used after drying it should be lightly dusted onto the surface before storage, and rinsed off before use.

The woman is invited to return to the clinic the following week with the cap *in situ* so that its correct position can be checked and size adjusted if necessary. The use of spermicides is then discussed in detail (section 8.3). The standard dose for effective protection is a 5 cm strip of jelly or cream smeared on each side of the dome. (i.e. 10 cm in all). If the spermicide produces an unacceptable leakage it is possible to dispense with the application on the undersurface at insertion as long as it is replaced by an application of foam. Whilst the cap should be inserted at a convenient time before intercourse, if more than three hours should elapse a pessary or foam should be inserted; a similar precaution should be taken when intercourse happens more than once. The cap should never be removed until at least six hours have elapsed since intercourse and may then be removed at any convenient time.

Caps can be purchased at any pharmaceutical chemist if the size is known, and they are also available from family planning clinics. It is usual to replace them annually and of course should they get damaged. If a woman loses more than 3.5 kg or gains a similar amount of weight the cap will need to be refitted. Spermicide is available from the same sources and there are a number of different preparations which allow for personal choice and sensitivity.

The efficiency of this method depends on an optimistic introduction, good teaching and good motivation. If the woman is not entirely satisfied or has any difficulty which she is afraid to reveal she will not use the cap regularly and unprotected intercourse will occur. It is important that nurses are sensitive to the ways in which women accept this type of contraception so that encouragement can be given when discussing any difficulties.

The cervical caps

The cervical caps are much smaller than the diaphragm and are less commonly used, but they have an important place in the barrier methods especially when there is a retroverted uterus with a forward thrusting cervix or when the vaginal wall muscle tone is poor. There are three types of cervical cap, the hollow-rimmed cervical cap, the vault cap and the vimule, which are identified in Figure 8.2.

The hollow-rimmed cervical cap
This cap is manufactured in four sizes ranging in 3 mm stages from 21 to 33 mm. It is thimble shaped and designed to fit snugly over a straight-sided cervix. First a speculum examination is necessary to assess the position and size of cervix which should be easily accessible and easily identified by the woman herself. When the correct size of cap has been selected it should be inserted by the family planning professional. This is accomplished by compressing the cap between finger and thumb and inserting it rim uppermost into the vagina where it can be guided over the cervix and pressed into position. The woman is then encouraged to feel it correctly positioned before removing it herself and reinserting it. When this has been successfully achieved the cap should be checked to make sure that it is in the correct position over the cervix. It is sometimes helpful to demonstrate, either with the fingers or on a model, how the cap fits over the cervix as this gives confidence and also explains how the suction needs to be released when taking the cap out. In normal use spermicide cream should be squeezed into the bowl of the cap before insertion and the outside smeared over as well whilst avoiding the rim itself. Some women find a pessary or stable foam easier to use on the external surface. Spermicide may need to be renewed in the same way as for the ordinary diaphragm and likewise the cervical cap should not be removed for at least six hours after intercourse. It should then be washed and stored as described earlier.

The vault cap
This cap clings to the vault of the vagina by suction. It is a shallow-domed rubber cap, and comes in five sizes arbitrarily numbered 1–5. The size is selected and the woman shown how to insert it as previously explained. The concave surface should be uppermost when the rim is compressed; it is then guided over the cervix with the index or third finger. The rim rests in the fornices and suction is created by pressing on the dome to exclude air once it is correctly positioned covering the cervix. The rim should never be smeared with cream or any lubricant as it weakens the suction action. The

vault cap is particularly useful when a woman's cervix is short and also where there are lax vaginal muscles or a small cystocoele.

The vimule cap
This cap is thimble shaped with a wider rim to promote strong suction. It is a hybrid of the cervical and vault caps already described and comes in three sizes: small, medium and large. This cap is especially useful when there is poor levator muscle tone in the vagina. It often has a thread attached to one side to assist removal. Spermicide cream needs to be applied inside and out but, once again, no cream should be used on the rim otherwise the suction action may be compromised. As an alternative a pessary or stable spermicide foam may be more easily used for protection on the external surface.

Correctly used, the barrier methods are efficient contraceptives with a pregnancy rate of 1.8/100 woman years. Failure is most common when the couple cannot anticipate their need for contraception and are unprepared. A growing popularity and widespread use illustrates their acceptability, with the added fringe benefits of reducing the risk of infection and having almost negligible side effects.

The contraceptive sponge

The sponge is made of soft polyurethane foam and looks like a small white doughnut with a dimple in the middle of the flattened surfaces. It is impregnated with spermicide and is indistinguishable from vaginal tissue. Prior to use, the sponge is thoroughly wetted and then squeezed before inserting it high up in the vagina, making sure that it quite covers the cervix. It provides a slow release mechanism for the spermicide, and the material of the sponge also acts as a sperm trap. It can be inserted whenever convenient, up to 24 hours prior to intercourse as the spermicide is slowly released for a total of 30 hours, but should remain in place for six hours after the last act of intercourse.

This is not a particularly reliable method of contraception having a failure rate of approximately 20% but like the sheath it has the definite advantage of not requiring medical supervision and being readily available. It is advisable, and overall results are likely to be better, when the user seeks advice on accurate insertion from her doctor or clinic.

8.3 SPERMICIDES

Spermicides in the form of jelly, cream, pessaries, aerosol foam, foaming tablets and dissolving film are all preparations currently available which contain substances lethal to sperm. It is difficult to believe that the forerunners of these sophisticated modern preparations which kill sperm almost immediately on contact were a long line of disagreeable and dubious spermicidal agents concocted by our ancestors in their attempts to secure the benefit of birth control. Brews of ox blood, tongues of linnets, cow dung, sponges soaked in wine, vinegar, honey, lemon juice or oil, fumigation and douching with soap and water were all earnestly prescribed to prevent conception, and many of the preparations must have been pretty obnoxious to handle. People practising family planning today are able to discuss with experts the merits of a wide variety of reliable spermicides according to preference, deciding on the smell and texture which are most agreeable to them. It is felt that this freedom of choice will eventually lead to more effective use of the chosen contraceptive.

The standard dose of jelly or cream is 10 cm (4 in.) squeezed from the tube. If this is applied to a diaphragm, 5 cm should be smeared on each side of the dome. When a cervical cap is used spermicide is squeezed into the bowl of the cap, but not on the rim as it will destroy suction.

With a pessary, it is recommended that this be inserted at a convenient time before intercourse, allowing 5–10 minutes for it to melt and disperse. Should intercourse occur again then the pessary needs to be repeated.

A foaming tablet must be dipped in water or moistened with saliva to achieve the foaming action before it is inserted, and like all pessaries it needs to be placed as high in the vagina as possible so that it is near the cervix.

Aerosol foam is marketed with a syringe and barrel applicator. The clear plastic barrel when fully filled contains the recommended dose. The full applicator is inserted until it reaches the top of the vagina and the contents are ejected any time up to an hour prior to intercourse. The foam is stable and remains effective for an hour but because of its physical properties it does not contribute much additional moisture to the vagina.

Spermicide film is available but cannot be relied upon as it can be difficult to insert correctly and the maximum dose of spermicide may not be in the optimum position where it is needed.

Some couples use spermicide without other methods of contraception. It cannot be recommended as a method with a high safety record, but it may be satisfactory especially later in life when the menopause is approaching and fertility of women is reduced. It has the added benefit of providing some lubrication when, if menopausal symptoms are present, the vagina may be a little dry. Because of the intended chemical destruction of sperm by chemically stripping off the outer cellular coat, the spermicides also have a useful part to play in killing the majority of bacteria and viruses which cause sexually transmitted disease. Most recently spermicides have been shown to have a positive effect in controlling the spread of the AIDS virus by killing it on contact.

9

Intrauterine devices

Intrauterine devices (IUDs) have been used as a method of contraception since the dawn of civilization, but they have only recently gained widespread popularity (Figures 9.1 and 9.2). The evolution of the present-day devices began in 1920 with Grafenberg's work. He first started using silkworm gut, then silver wire in various forms of rings and springs so that the device stayed in place. His most successful attempt was with a silver coiled wire which was commercially manufactured in 1928, but unfortunately pelvic infection became associated with the fitting of IUDs and as antibiotics were yet to be discovered the publicity aroused was such that the idea was not a resounding success.

At about the same time in Japan entirely independent work was being carried out by Ota, who started with the same silkworm gut rings and also used other flexible materials. It was quite natural for him to progress to using plastics once they were developed and readily available, and by 1959 a number of different workers were designing and trying spiral devices, loops and all sorts of shapes easily manufactured from the newly invented plastic. Each of these different designs tried to fulfil the criteria of easy, painless introduction with high retention rates in the uterus and low risk pregnancy. Of these original designs the Lippe's loop remains in use.

Shield-like shapes were tested and were highly successful with some women. Although the retention rate was high they were difficult to insert and had a tendency to upset the periods. The Dalkon shield, though effective in preventing pregnancy and remaining *in situ* when other devices would have been extruded, was given adverse publicity in 1978 when it was reported that accidental pregnancies occurring with this device had a risk of

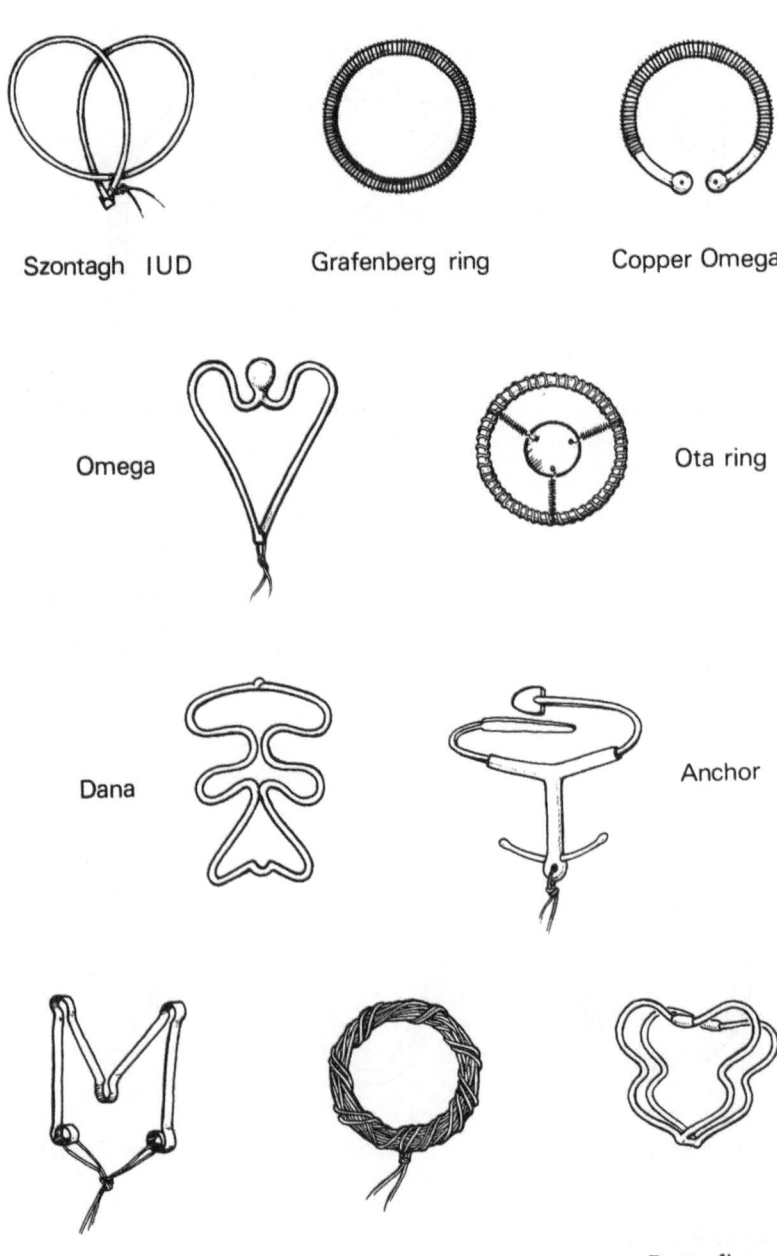

Szontagh IUD   Grafenberg ring   Copper Omega

Omega

Ota ring

Dana

Anchor

M 213   Zipper ring   Butterfly

Figure 9.1 Historical interest.

Margulies spiral   Birnberg bow   Soonawala Y

Soonawala IUD   Dalkon Shield – nulliparous   Dalkon Shield – multiparous

Hall-Stone ring   Antigon   Winged Antigon

Figure 9.1 *continued.*

septic mid-trimester abortion. Although these reports were not confirmed, the device was withdrawn by the manufacturers because of litigation, and doctors were advised to remove any

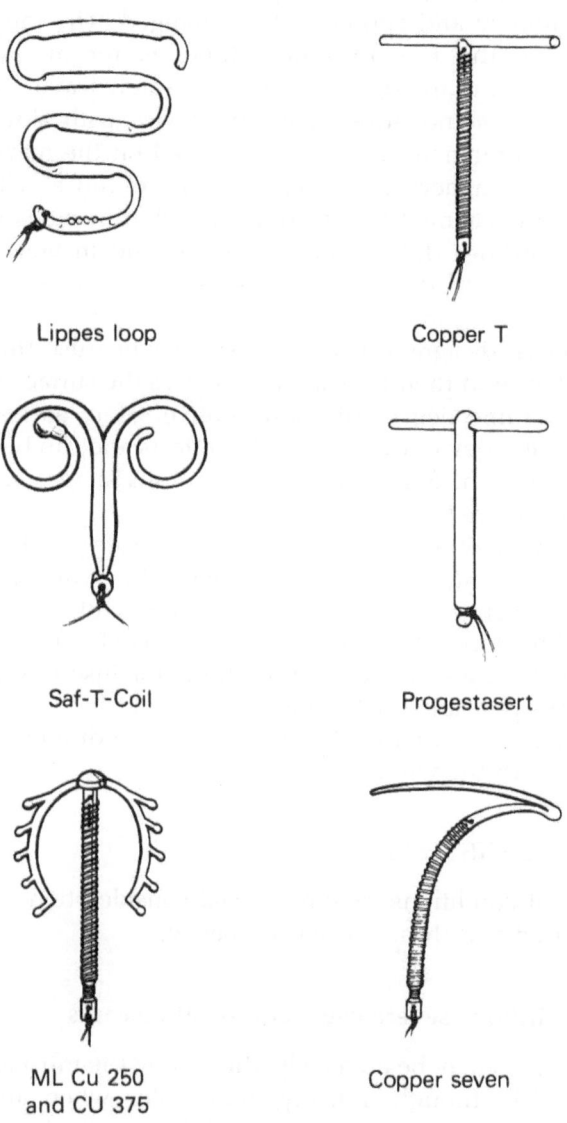

Lippes loop

Copper T

Saf-T-Coil

Progestasert

ML Cu 250
and CU 375

Copper seven

Figure 9.2 Recent designs in intrauterine devices.

which were still in use. The Saf-T-Coil was evolved during the 1950s and this device was found to have a good retention rate and is still being used by some doctors.

Plastic devices without any copper wire may remain in the uterus indefinitely and should not be changed. The longer they remain in use the less likelihood there is for an accidental pregnancy to occur, and older women may safely leave them until a year after the menopause. A plastic device with slow-release progesterone contained in its stem appeared on the market for a short time. Pregnancy rates were similar to those with other devices, but the claimed benefit of a reduction in menstrual loss and dysmenorrhoea did not always occur, and in view of high manufacturing cost the device was not a success and was withdrawn from the market.

Most modern designs can now be smaller because the copper wire wound around their thin stems increases the surface area and provides the same degree of contraceptive safety as something larger. A smaller device causes less side effects and can be used by nulliparous women. For details of the various shapes which are available see Figure 9.2.

As with other methods of contraception, the safety and reliability of this method must be discussed with the woman and an explanation given about the practical aspects of inserting the device into the uterus. A comprehensive history should be taken to ensure that there are no contraindications for inserting an IUD. The doctor responsible for the insertion should have this history available when he discusses the advantages and disadvantages of the method with the woman.

9.1 MEDICAL HISTORY

Some medical conditions require special consideration before an IUD is inserted and these are set out below.

Cardiac conditions, severe chest and renal diseases

These conditions may be adversely affected by the introduction of infection which, though unlikely, may occur when an IUD is inserted into the uterine cavity providing systemic entry for bacteria. Specialist advice is necessary before deciding on this method of contraception.

Anaemia

The possibility of menorrhagia, or even slightly heavier periods than usual, may exacerbate this condition, coupled with a slight risk of infection which would be difficult for the individual to combat. Until the cause can be diagnosed and treated an IUD could worsen the condition.

Thromboembolic conditions

If these conditions necessitate the use of anticoagulant therapy, the insertion of an IUD may cause problems by increasing the menstrual blood loss or by causing intermenstrual bleeding.

Epilepsy

There is a potential risk of epileptics having a fit at the time of IUD insertion and staff should be prepared for this to happen. It is preferable for an expert and dextrous doctor to carry out the procedure.

Steroid therapy

If any condition exists which necessitates steroid treatment the possibility of the drug masking pelvic infection and the risk of the IUD provoking it needs to be considered.

9.2 GYNAECOLOGICAL HISTORY

Dysmenorrhoea or menorrhagia

An accurate menstrual history will determine whether these conditions already exist or have ever been experienced. Although neither are direct contraindications, both conditions may worsen somewhat in the presence of an IUD and should be carefully supervised.

Post-coital insertion

It should be made quite clear to the woman from the start that an established pregnancy is seldom disturbed by the insertion of a device, but if there is any doubt about the last menstrual period it is better to delay the insertion until pregnancy is diagnosed or the period arrives. Some women unjustly believe that IUDs are inserted without careful investigation and that the insertion will cause an early abortion. A device inserted in the five days following unprotected intercourse will act something akin to the 'morning after' pill, but the difference is that it is being used before any period is missed or a pregnancy established.

Irregular vaginal bleeding

This is a contraindication and a diagnosis must be made and treatment carried out before any insertion is attempted. The possibility of a threatened abortion should be explored as a possible cause of the intermittent bleeding.

Abnormalities of the uterine cavity

Fibroids may alter the shape of the uterine cavity (Figure 9.3) and make insertion and retention of a device more difficult. A bicornuate uterus or one with a small septum may also cause difficulties and if the device remains in the cavity it may become distorted and cause pain and menorrhagia. In extreme cases pregnancy may occur.

Pelvic inflammatory disease

A history of this condition must be treated if it is suspected, before insertion of the device. The woman with a past history of pelvic infection requires very careful assessment to make sure that no residual infection exists, as this can be precipitated to cause a fresh outbreak of infection when irritated by the presence of a foreign body.

Cervical and vaginal discharge

A history of irritating or purulent and offensive vaginal discharge should always be brought to the attention of the doctor. It is helpful where this facility is possible to take swabs for culture and sensitivity, and the cervix needs to be particularly well cleaned before insertion of an IUD where this is considered to be without hazard. If the cervical discharge appears purulent it is considerably

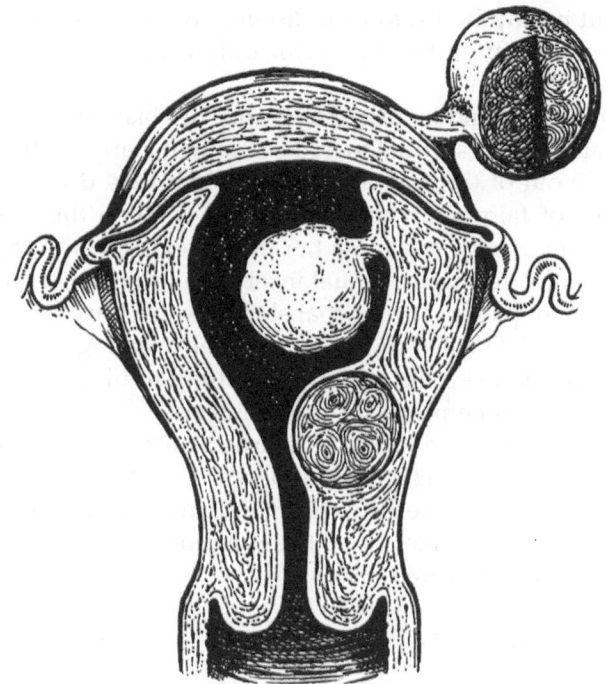

Figure 9.3 Fibroids distorting the uterine cavity.

wiser to delay insertion until after the specific treatment has been completed.

Old cervical damage

Old lacerations of the cervix caused by childbirth (even when repaired) or a history of cone biopsy may give rise to problems both with retention of the device within the uterine cavity and by increasing risk of creating a false passage whilst trying to negotiate the cervical canal.

9.3 IUD INSERTION

Once the type of IUD has been decided upon, the procedure should be explained to the woman and insertion of the device then carried out promptly. Prolonged discussion and a long wait before being seen and fitted by the doctor only contribute to mounting anxiety and tension.

The woman should be asked to empty her bladder and undress appropriately. It is essential to make sure that if any clothes are left on they are out of the way and loose so that they do not increase the chance of fainting. The nurse needs to keep the woman as relaxed as possible by engaging her in conversation and remaining in close contact during the actual insertion of the device, watching for any signs of pain or fear so that she can warn the doctor. It is no easier to fit an IUD when the woman is menstruating and it may be unsatisfactory to keep her waiting for fitting until her next period as she could become pregnant in the interval.

The chosen device and a set of instruments need to be prepared (Table 9.1). In most clinics the packs are already sterile and prepared by a central sterile supply department, but a few clinics still manage with sterilizers, and the equipment will be prepared in advance and kept covered.

Table 9.1 Equipment for insertion of an IUD

1 × spencer wells
1 × pair scissors
1 × sponge holding forceps
1 × allis tissue forceps or tenaculum
1 × cusco's speculum
1 × uterine sound
1 × kidney dish
2 × small dishes for swabs and disinfectant
1 × clean sanitary towel
2 × sterile towels (optional)

Don't forget the device! (and a spare one)

In order to increase the ease with which the fitting is made the doctor and nurse must take every care to conduct the proceedings in a confident and reassuring manner, so that the woman is as relaxed and confident as possible. (One unfortunate woman commented that she had requested an IUD to be fitted at another clinic and she had left without it when she observed the doctor concentrating on reading the instructions for insertion!) Personal privacy needs to be guarded before the woman is positioned on the couch either on her back with her knees bent and legs abducted or in the left lateral with both her knees partially drawn up. A good light source is essential which can be directed into the vagina. After a bimanual examination to assess the size and position of the uterus, a cusco's speculum is lubricated and inserted into the vagina, and the cervix is exposed. If cervical cytology is required, now is the time to take a smear prior to cleaning the cervix with a swab soaked in savlon or some suitable disinfectant.

Most operators place a tenaculum on the anterior part of the cervix to align the angle of the uterine cavity with the cervical canal. The uterine sound is then passed through the cervix and the length and direction of the cavity is noted. The device is taken from its sterile wrapping and folded into the introducer ready for insertion; this should occur without delay so that the plastic does not lose its shape and become distorted. Techniques for the introduction of each device differ slightly, the general aim being to insert the device into the cavity of the uterus whilst it is temporarily straightened. Once inside it is released to take up its original shape which is designed to retain it in the correct position. No undue pressure must be used as it is possible to perforate the uterus. The whole device, including the lowest part of the stem, must lie well within the cavity for it to be totally effective, and no part of the stem should extrude through the cervix. After placing the device in the correct position, the monofilament nylon thread is shortened with care being taken not to cut it so short that it either forms a prickly spike or, worse still, disappears altogether into the uterus. On the other hand it must not be left so long that it becomes intrusive to the woman, and the correct length is probably about 2 cm so that it can comfortably curl up into the fornices. The excess thread can be handed to the woman so that she can recognize the consistency and identify it when she makes her routine checks as recommended after each period has finished. A sanitary towel or panty liner should be offered to the woman in case of slight spotting from the tenaculum where it punctured the cervix. On removing the speculum care should be taken to ensure that the thread of the IUD does not become trapped in the jaws, causing the device to become dislodged. A correctly positioned IUD is shown in Figure 9.4.

No woman should be allowed to hurry away from the clinic after an IUD insertion. Any immediate cramps generally disappear within a few hours and rarely cause much trouble, but there may

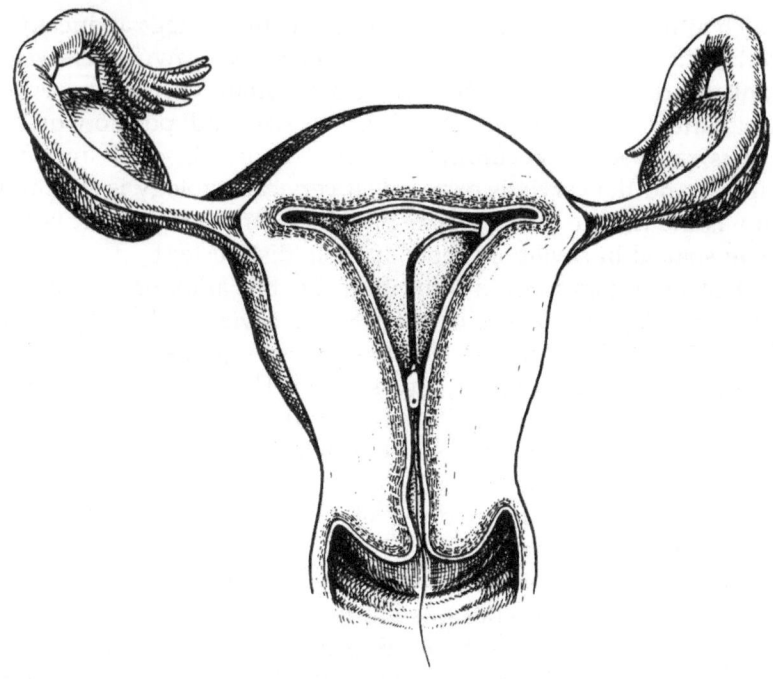

Figure 9.4 Intrauterine device (copper seven) in place.

be a delayed tendency to faint and this is upsetting not only to the woman herself but also to all the others who witness it whilst they are awaiting their own turn. Some women are very confident and relaxed, but this is not always the case. A few may be very nervous and tense and sheer anxiety may lead to faintness and nausea. Others experience considerable uterine cramp and will be grateful for analgesic tablets to relieve the pain before dressing. Sometimes the cramping pain may be very severe and though this is rare the woman may suffer from shock. For all these reasons it may be best to ask the woman to rest awhile before departure.

Advice after insertion of IUD

It is wise to show the woman the actual device so that she knows what has been inserted. It may also be helpful for her to feel the stem so that she can recognize it by touch if it extrudes from the cervix. If this happens she should return to the clinic at once as the device is not effective unless it is in the correct position within the uterine cavity. In this circumstance the device needs to be removed and a new one inserted. The woman should know that this contraceptive method is immediately effective and will continue to be so until it is removed, expelled or requires changing after the date of expiry. If the device is plain plastic it will not require changing, whilst devices with copper wire wound around the stems are at present changed every 3–5 years. It is therefore important that a note is made of the nature of the device fitted, and that the woman herself knows how long the device will protect her. The IUD is said to have a failure rate of 2–3/100 woman years.

The woman should be asked to return to the clinic if she has any complaints and she should do so if there is bleeding which continues for more than 24 hours or if pain occurs which is not relieved by mild analgesia. Advice about who to contact and how should be provided especially outside normal clinic hours. The first few periods are likely to be heavier than usual and may be associated with dysmenorrhoea until the device settles in. If the woman usually uses tampons this is quite acceptable as they are unlikely to dislodge the device. The most likely time for the device to be expelled is during the first period following insertion, so an appointment should be made six weeks later to check that it remains in place and that the threads are visualized during speculum examination.

Before leaving the clinic the woman should be given a letter to her general practitioner informing him about insertion details and identifying the type of IUD used.

9.4 IUD COMPLICATIONS

Fainting and vasovagal attacks

These occur occasionally, but they are rare and can be minimized with good clinic management. The woman should be dealt with efficiently and seen without undue waiting. Good clinic ventilation and a friendly and relaxed atmosphere reduce the number of incidents. Should a woman faint she should be laid flat on her back with her legs raised, unless there is any difficulty with maintaining an airway, when she is better placed lying on one or other side. Tight clothing, especially around the neck, needs to be loosened, and if the clinic is warm fanning with anything which comes to hand may be helpful. It is important to make and note general observations of pulse, respiration and colour and if recovery is in any way delayed to estimate the blood pressure. The importance of an unobstructed airway cannot be overstressed.

It is rare for a woman's condition not to improve swiftly and spontaneously but if there is a delay she should be given atropine sulphate 0.6 mg intravenously. In a few cases it is necessary to remove the device and if it is still decided to use this method of contraception it is wise to select a smaller device and introduce it whilst the woman has a general anaesthetic. It is always wise to keep other causes of sudden collapse in mind; occasionally epileptic fits or more rarely coronary thrombosis can be the cause.

Cramp and bleeding

It is not uncommon for dysmenorrhoea to accompany the fitting of a device. Most women recover quickly and only a few need mild analgesia. If the cramp and pain are severe it may be necessary to give mefenamic acid (Ponstan) and the woman should be encouraged to rest at the clinic until she feels better.

Bleeding may occur from the site of the tenaculum, but it is rarely heavy. Irregular bleeding and pain may be effectively dealt with by removal of the device and insertion of a smaller one. If severe bleeding occurs and blood clots are reported the woman needs to be referred to a gynaecological department as occasionally this may be due to spontaneous abortion.

Expulsion

This may occur without the woman being aware of the expulsion until she feels for the threads and is then unable to locate them. Sometimes pain and bleeding accompany expulsion and for this reason every woman reporting these symptoms should have a speculum examination to see whether the threads or part of the device are visible.

Uterine perforation

This is a rare but ever present risk. It occurs at insertion and is usually accompanied by abdominal or pelvic pain possibly associated with shock. Occasionally there are no noticeable symptoms at the time and the woman returns at a later date with problems. The accident is more likely to happen with post-natal and post-abortion cases where the uterus is soft and more easily penetrated. It may also occur if the angle of the uterus is markedly anteverted or retroverted when the device is pushed through the myometrium in error, particularly if a tenaculum is not used during the insertion of a slim device like a copper seven.

If the woman has been using oral contraception for several years and more than five years have elapsed since her last child was born, the cervix may be much tougher making the insertion of an IUD more difficult and it is the extra pressure required which can result in perforation. Perforation should be suspected if the threads of the device are not visible following insertion or if the uterine sound or introducer appears to go too far into the uterus. If the uterus has been perforated arrangements must be made for immediate admission to hospital where a gynaecologist can retrieve the device from the abdominal cavity and if necessary repair the uterine damage.

The lost thread

The whereabouts of the IUD should be established. A gently manipulated probe may bring the thread into sight; if not arrangements must be made for an ultrasonic scan to determine the position of the device and make sure that it has not been expelled.

Infection

Statistics indicate only a very slight increase in infection rates of women fitted with IUDs over those using other contraceptive methods. The IUD certainly provides no protection from sexually transmitted infection as the barrier methods do. If the woman is carefully examined and gives an accurate history before she has an IUD inserted it is possible to minimize the risks by treating existing infection first. However, low grade infection if missed can flare up in the presence of a foreign body in the uterine cavity. If infection does occur it generally responds well to treatment. Occasionally it is necessary to remove the device, treat the infection and then re-introduce the device at a later time if requested. If this is necessary, adequate alternative contraception should be arranged. Pregnancy at the time of uterine infection could produce dangerous consequences.

In certain parts of the world the escalation of claims against the manufacturers which are difficult to disprove have caused many IUDs to be withdrawn in specific localities. However in those places where sanity prevails this reliable and safe method of contraception continues to be available.

Pregnancy with IUD *in situ*

The statistics show a pregnancy rate of 2–3 per hundred woman years. If the pregnancy is allowed to continue the IUD is often expelled with the placenta during the third stage of labour. It remains outside the amniotic sac and never comes into contact with the fetus.

The incidence of spontaneous abortion where there is an IUD *in situ* is only slightly higher than the average rate of abortion which is approximately 1 in 10 for any pregnancy. Although there are many women who seek termination when this method has failed, there are some who wish to continue the pregnancy. There are two approaches which are equally valid; one is to leave everything alone and not disrupt the uterine equilibrium; the other involves removing the device at the first opportunity if the threads are visible. This removes the fear of ascending infection and mid-trimester abortion but may risk causing slight haemorrhage.

Ectopic pregnancy associated with IUD

Those who use IUDs are no more likely to develop an ectopic pregnancy than anyone else. But as this method does not prevent ovulation, occasional fertilization is possible with the risk of tubal pregnancy the same as normal. If a woman complains of pregnancy symptoms or has pelvic pain, an ectopic pregnancy should be suspected and investigated.

9.5 ADVANTAGES OF THE IUD

This method of contraception is very acceptable to many women. It is immediately effective and requires only the motivation to arrange an appointment for insertion. Once it has been checked six weeks following insertion the clinic visits are annual. It allows a completely spontaneous lifestyle and gives the woman complete protection until its removal. It is rarely felt by the partner and in no way interferes with his spontaneity or sensation. Ovulation is not affected or suppressed. The insertion is quick and easily available, and fertility returns rapidly after the device is removed so that the pattern of pregnancies can be fairly accurately planned.

9.6 REMOVAL OF IUD

If an alternative method of contraception is contemplated it should be initiated before the IUD is removed to allow the woman to adjust to the new method without leaving her unprotected. The menstrual cycle should also be estimated and if the request for removal is at the time of ovulation it would be wise to defer it for a week to avoid the possibility of conception if there are active sperm in the reproductive tract.

In order to remove a device it is necessary to have available a vaginal speculum (preferably bivalve), spencer wells forceps and a good light. After locating the thread, steady traction will bring the device out quite easily with very little discomfort. On rare occasions the device may have become misshapen or wedged into the myometrium or cervical canal and will cause pain when removal is attempted. It is therefore advisable for a doctor or nurse who is trained in family planning to remove the device although there are a few women who do it for themselves. Some women require a general anaesthetic for insertion as well as removal and it is obviously preferable in these cases to use a device which needs less frequent changing.

10

Physiological methods of avoiding pregnancy

10.1 THE SAFE PERIOD

The safe period (also known as the rhythm method or periodic abstinence) is approved by Roman Catholics as the only acceptable method of controlling the size of the family. In order to use this method effectively it is necessary to estimate as accurately as possible when ovulation is likely to occur and avoid intercourse during this time. This is not the safest method of birth control because irregularities in the menstrual cycle occur in most women making calculation of ovulation inaccurate. If it is the couple's inclination to use this method, then every encouragement should be given to help them in assessing the safe period as accurately as possible: in this way many pregnancies will be avoided.

Calculation of ovulation

Certain hormonal changes occurring during the menstrual cycle help to estimate the time of ovulation by causing recognizable alterations in the woman's body (Figure 10.1). These methods can be used either together or singly but if only one method is used it will tend to be less accurate.

The calendar method
This method requires a record of the onset of periods in the preceding six months. From this record, which should be constantly updated, the details of the shortest and longest cycles are taken. Ovulation is said to occur between 12 and 16 days, with an average of 14 days, before the onset of the next period. When variation in the span of the cycle is studied it is possible using these dates to estimate the unsafe days and avoid intercourse during this time

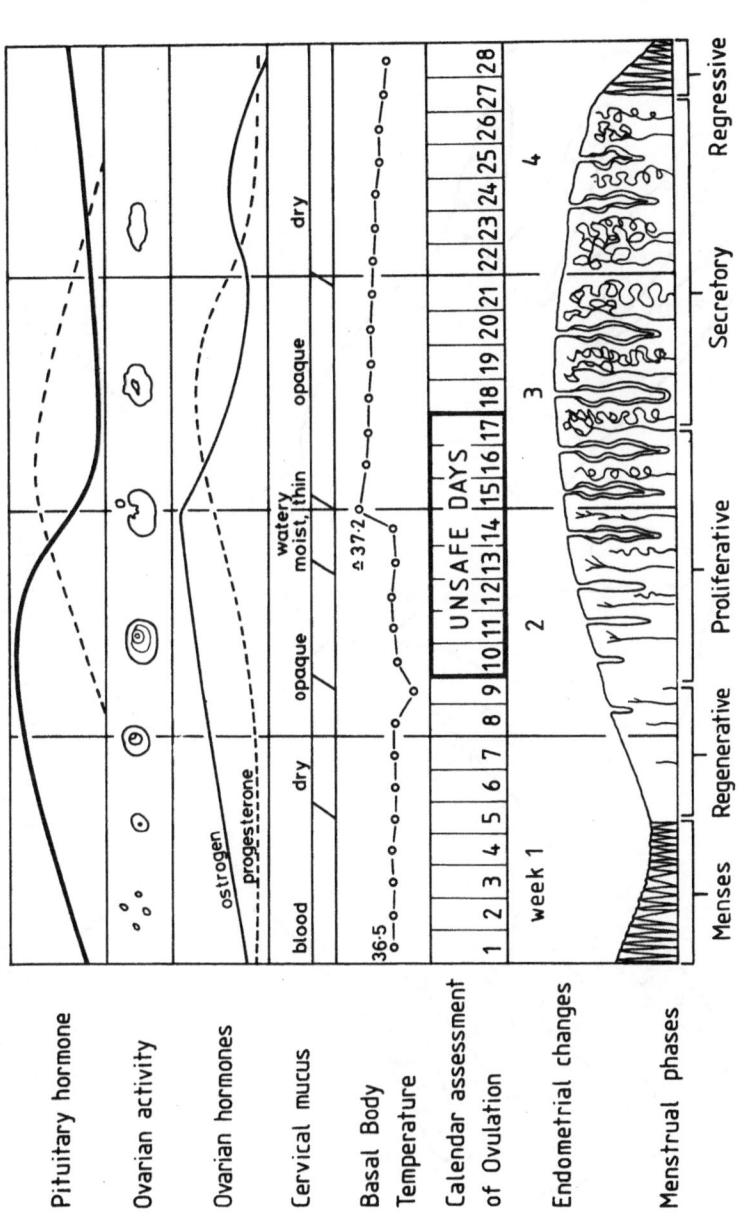

Figure 10.1 Physiological changes in the menstrual cycle in conjunction with physiological methods of birth control.

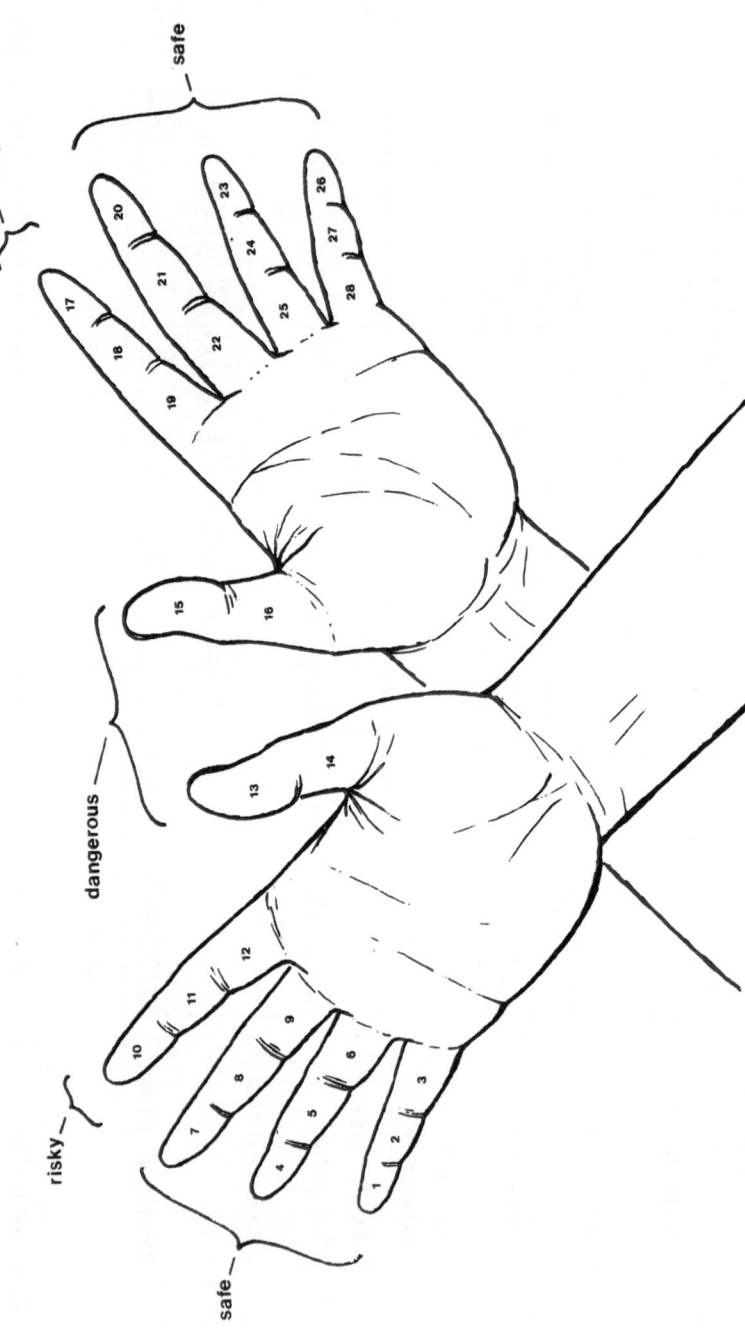

Figure 10.2 The safe period. A very simple method of demonstrating and dividing a 28 day month into periods of relative safety and absolute danger. When couples choose to use the safe period all days prior to day 20 should be considered a risk.

Table 10.1 Calculating the unsafe days of the menstrual cycle

Length of shortest cycle in days	First unsafe day after start of period	Length of longest cycle in days	Last unsafe day after start of period
20	1	20	9
21	2	21	10
22	3	22	11
23	4	23	12
24	5	24	13
25	6	25	14
26	7	26	15
27	8	27	16
28	9	28	17
29	10	29	18
30	11	30	19
31	12	31	20
32	13	32	21
33	14	33	22
34	15	34	23
35	16	35	24
36	17	36	25

Example:
During the previous six months a woman has had menstrual cycles lasting respectively 27, 25, 28, 26, 30 and 28 days.
1. The shortest cycle is 25 days which reading from the chart shows day 6 to be the first unsafe day.
2. The longest cycle is 30 days which reading from the chart shows day 19 to be the last unsafe day.
3. The predicted unsafe period therefore lasts from day 6 to day 19 of any month if all eventualities are to be covered.
4. Subsequent cycles are taken into account each month to keep the intermediate six months as the basis of calculation.

(Figure 10.2 and Table 10.1). The unsafe days are the 3 days before and the two days after ovulation. This ensures that the sperm which usually live for up to 3 days have perished before ovulation, and that the ovum, which may live for up to 48 hours, will have become defunct before intercourse is resumed.

Where the variations in the cycle are slight this method may be effective and acceptable; unfortunately when the cycles vary in length estimating the unsafe days for both the shortest and longest cycles will meant that long periods of abstinence will be necessary. As an example, if a woman's record indicates that her shortest cycle is 24 days and her longest cycle is 34 days, the first unsafe day will be day 5, just after her period has finished, and it will not be safe for her to resume intercourse until after day 23.

Body temperature
This method depends on noticing the small but sustained rise in the basal body temperature occurring when there is an increase in the progesterone level which results from ovulation. The woman has to take her temperature before rising each morning and record it on a chart. When a rise of temperature is evident it suggests that ovulation has taken place and as a precaution intercourse should be avoided for 24 hours. However, it is not until this temperature rise has been maintained for a further 24 hours that ovulation can be confirmed, so that on a practical basis abstinence after ovulation is necessary for 2 or 3 days. The temperature rise is maintained until the end of the cycle. Unfortunately this method gives **no pre-ovulatory warning** so sperm which may have been deposited in the female reproductive tract could fertilize the ovum. It should be borne in mind too that a rise in temperature may be due to the presence of pyrexia provoking illness.

The mucus method
Changes in cervical mucus as described in Chapter 2 can be helpful in estimating the progress of the cycle. When circulating levels of oestrogen are high the mucus has a thin watery texture with considerable stretchability in its threads (good spinbarkeit). This is an indication that the mucus can be easily penetrated by sperm on their way through the cervix at a time when ovulation is occurring. This change gives some pre-ovulatory warning and with practice a woman can learn to test the changes in the mucus. Local infection causing changes in vaginal secretions may however contribute to less accurate results.

Home predictor kits
There are a number of commercially available kits which accurately test for the presence of the LH (luteinizing hormone) surge which precedes ovulation. A simple procedure makes use of an indicator which changes colour when in contact with urine. The manufacturers' instructions are easily understood and simple to follow. Because they are not cheap it is unlikely that the kits would be used every month but they are a useful adjunct to other physiological

methods to confirm the accuracy of the routine method(s) of prediction.

10.2 COITUS INTERRUPTUS (WITHDRAWAL)

When using this method the man withdraws his penis from the vagina just before ejaculation. The Book of Genesis states that Onan spilt his seed upon the ground to prevent fertilization of his brother's wife (38:9). This must surely be one of the earliest references to contraception! A more modern expression referring to this method of family planning is 'being careful'. It is difficult to know how many couples use this method today. In 1969 Peel recorded that 44% of couples had used it at some time and that for 21% it was the current method. It does necessitate concentration and may cause some sexual frustration if orgasm is not achieved. Those who use it regularly are unlikely to come into contact with health professionals unless a psycho-sexual problem or an unplanned pregnancy occurs. As the man becomes older it may be more difficult to achieve the necessary control and the woman may then seek advice about another method. Coitus interruptus is not renowned for its safety and carries a pregnancy rate of approximately 20/100 woman years. However, it is better than making no effort to control reproduction at all and may work well for some couples.

11

Sterilization

Sterilization is surgical alteration of the reproductive anatomy in the male or female in order to prevent conception: it should generally be regarded as irreversible. Because of the permanent nature of this particular contraceptive technique it is essential that health professionals are able to provide accurate information and adequate counselling so that those seeking advice are correctly informed about the suitability of the method. It is not unusual to find that people have irrational ideas about the effect of sterilization on their sexual function, and whilst some men may mistakenly fear that their sexual activity may be diminished, women are not without their fair share of apprehensions. In some cases the couple may expect an unrealistic improvement in sexual relationships. It is therefore important that the reason for the couple asking for sterilization is fully discussed.

There are no hard and fast rules about who is and who is not suitable for sterilization. Of course guidelines can be drawn, but familiarity with techniques and experience in counselling will generally minimize errors of judgement. The most important considerations are marital stability, family size, and for how long the procedure has been contemplated. The choice of who to sterilize may be dictated by medical considerations and therefore it is important to collate a full medical history from each partner before the final decision is made. Age should also be taken into account because where more years of reproductive life remain, a greater possibility exists for the development of doubt. This is less of a potential risk in women who naturally conclude childbearing a little before the menopause, whereas men continue to produce sperm long after they have reached their dotage.

The question of reversibility sometimes arises, and whilst reconstruction of the fallopian tube is occasionally possible there are many disappointments. A successful reversal of vasectomy is more likely if the period of sterility has been short, because the formation of anti-sperm antibodies increases with time reducing the number of sperm that are produced. If the couple are not prepared to make a positive decision they should not be forced into committing themselves at this stage and more time needs to be made available for discussion.

11.1 FEMALE STERILIZATION

This involves bilateral occlusion of the fallopian tubes with or without division and has been historically labelled as tubal ligation. A number of different methods are available which are usually carried out under general anaesthetic. Access to the abdomen may be made through a traditional skin incision or via a laparoscope which is inserted through a minute cut in the lower edge of the umbilicus. Continuity of the tubes may be interrupted by division and ligation, bipolar diathermization, or the permanent application of some form of specialized clip or sialastic ring (Figure 11.1).

Women often ask what happens to the ovum each month when it cannot pass along the fallopian tube because of the surgical interruption. The simple answer is that it is so minute that it is

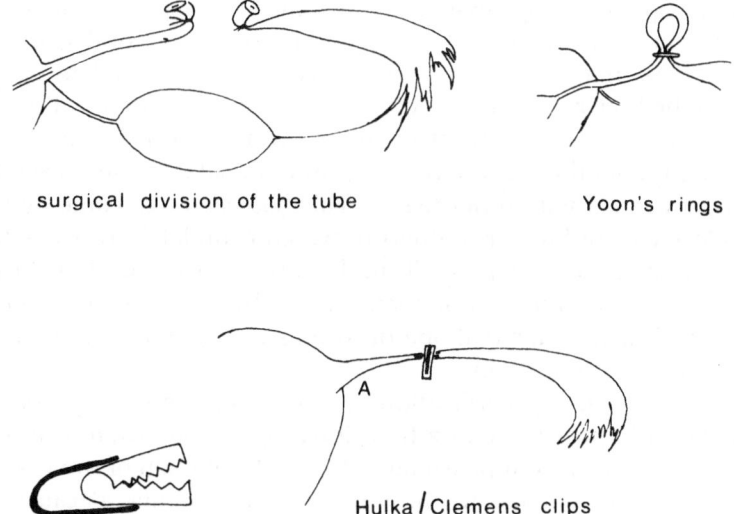

surgical division of the tube   Yoon's rings

Hulka / Clemens clips

Figure 11.1 Sterilization methods.

readily absorbed in the remaining portion of the tube or the peritoneal cavity.

Laparoscopic sterilization

Laparoscopy allows intra-abdominal visualization of the pelvic organs through a thin metal tube containing an optical system. It has become increasingly popular because the scars when healed are scarcely seen and the time spent in hospital can be as short as one day.

The patient is usually given a general anaesthetic which produces complete muscle relaxation. The bladder is emptied by catheterization and a sound is passed into the uterine cavity and left there for positioning the uterus later in the operation. A measured volume of carbon dioxide is injected into the abdominal cavity through a Verrey's needle which has a spring loaded guard over its sharp point to prevent bowel injury. About 2 litres of gas are necessary to raise the abdomen in a dome. The patient is then tilted head downwards so that the bowels fall away from the operating zone in the pelvis, and a trocar and cannula are inserted through the umbilical incision. The trocar is then removed and the laparoscope is passed through the cannula. A fibreoptic lighting system provides clear illumination of the pelvic organs.

When an operating laparoscope is available it is possible to avoid further puncture of the abdomen. Otherwise a second trocar is inserted so that specialized forceps can be introduced to manipulate the tube and carry out the chosen method of sterilization. In the early days the fallopian tubes were burnt by ordinary diathermy, but there was a risk of unintentional damage caused by indirect contact with other tissue. This has been overcome by the development of bipolar diathermy which completely restricts the effect to the tissue grasped within the forceps. Methods have been developed to occlude the fallopian tubes by local pressure; these include sialastic rings (Fallope or Yoon's rings) and clips (Hulka–Clemens or Filshie clips).

Anyone expecting sterilization by laparoscopy must be prepared to accept the possibility of a traditional operation. There is also a small but ever-present possibility of the introduction of the trocars causing some damage to intra-abdominal contents. Because of these reservations all concerned with the operation must make it clear that although it is perfectly possible in the uncomplicated laparoscopy to return home within 24 hours, it is advisable to be prepared to stay longer as up to 1 in 100 patients may have to have a laparotomy. This depends on the skill and expertise of the operator as well as on the normality of the pelvic anatomy. As individuals requiring sterilization are likely to have young families it is essential that they understand the last point so that arrangements for looking after the children during the mother's extended absence are prearranged.

Tubal ligation

This form of sterilization is preferred by some gynaecologists as it has slightly less risk of failure. There are many small variations between techniques, but most conform to the well proven Pomeroy's operation. This operation requires a general anaesthetic and consists of removing a small segment of fallopian tube and ligating the cut ends. There are some other popular techniques and it is quite possible to apply clips or sialastic rings through a small horizontal scar hidden in the pubic hair. This technique is known as minilaparotomy.

In the puerperium, following the birth of a baby, it is possible to make a small incision in the lower edge of the umbilicus and find the fallopian tubes nearby because of the enlarged uterus. The risks of venous thrombosis and pulmonary embolism from operations performed in the puerperium are above average and only justify this approach to sterilization in a few selected cases. The majority are better left for laparoscopic sterilization after six weeks or more. It is possible to reduce the extent of the surgery by utilizing the laparoscope, but it requires skilled handling owing to the enlarged uterus and in any case does not reduce the amount of anaesthesia necessary.

11.2 MALE STERILIZATION

Vasectomy

The vas deferens convey the sperm from the testes to storage glands known as seminal vesicles which are situated just below the bladder. Each vas travels upwards in the spermatic cord and passes from the scrotum along the inguinal canal on its own side to enter the abdomen through the internal inguinal ring. Division of this duct may be performed anywhere along its length, but in practice it is more convenient to operate in the scrotum. Once bilaterally divided it is impossible for any further sperm formed in the testes to be ejaculated by the male during intercourse. There is, however, an interval during which previously produced sperm are still present in the duct system. These will be gradually eliminated by ejaculation.

Whilst the operation of vasectomy may be performed under general anaesthesia it is usually carried out under local anaesthesia as an out-patient procedure. The men are told to arrive at the clinic having bathed and shaved off their pubic hair. The scrotum is prepared for operation and a local anaesthetic is then injected into the scrotal skin. Two small incisions are usually required. The spermatic cords are individually exposed and a pair of clamps are applied so that a small segment can be removed. This is sent for histological examination to confirm that the structure has been divided and its removal leaves a gap between the cut ends which are less likely to join together. The clamped ends of the tubes are firmly tied with a slowly dissolving polymer suture and when released will spring apart as a safeguard against recanalization. A check is made to discover any small bleeding points and these are tied or coagulated since otherwise they might lead to the formation of an haematoma which can become gross and very painful. With one side completed a similar technique is required for the other side. Some surgeons operate through a single scrotal incision but this necessitates puncturing the scrotal septum with further risk of haematoma. At the end of the operation the skin incisions are closed and the wounds covered with a plastic spray dressing. The scrotum is then well protected by wearing an athletic or medical scrotal support.

Following the operation instructions are given to avoid strenuous exercise for a day or two. The man will be more comfortable wearing firm underpants to provide support for the scrotum. If the scrotum begins to swell, or shows bruising, it is necessary for the man to seek advice from his general practitioner or from the surgeon who carried out the operation, for should an haematoma develop the scrotum can become grossly distended and extremely painful. Fortunately this complication occurs in less than 4% of cases.

Following the operation, specimens of semen are sent for analysis at intervals of six weeks or as convenient and thereafter as necessary until two consecutive specimens show no sperm at all. Following the second result the operation may be declared successful. It is important to stress that abstinence from intercourse is unhelpful as ejaculation is necessary to clear the sperm reservoir, but it is important that adequate safeguards are taken against unintended pregnancy whilst waiting for the all clear.

A small number of operations fail, either due to reanastomosis or recanalization of the vas or because there is a secondary system which has gone unrecognized. After the operation the man will have no idea that the sperm element is missing from his semen as it only forms a minute part of the ejaculated fluid. The greater part of the ejaculate consists of secretions from the prostate gland which are intended to provide nourishment for the sperm. No difference is therefore noted in the quantity of semen produced.

12

Cervical cytology

Screening for cervical cancer is now an established service for sexually active women. The incidence of abnormal changes in the cervix has risen and this fact, which has had considerable publicity, has increased the demand for screening services. Unfortunately there is still a substantial undetected incidence of cervical neoplastic disease amongst those women who shy away from preventive medical care. Factors which seem to influence vulnerability of women to the disease include those who started having intercourse at an early age or having a number of different partners. In the latter case even if the woman has only had a single sexual partner she may be at risk if the man has had multiple relationships.

The possible viral origins of the disease should be considered when there is a history of wart virus or herpes genitalis. Barrier methods of contraception may have a positive role in reducing risk. Women over 35 and those of lower socio-economic status need to be identified by the nurse and particularly encouraged to have regular cervical smears.

Before specifically considering the screening programme for cervical cytology it may be helpful to note some of the criteria which should be met before any sort of screening programme is established.

12.1 SCREENING CRITERIA

The method of screening must be accurate enough to define the disease clearly and avoid frequent false positive or negative results. The method of testing must be acceptable to the public and should never involve procedures which produce more risk to the patient than the disease! There must be adequate facilities for obtaining the specimen and performing the laboratory testing so that reports are produced within a reasonable period. There must be staff and facilities to investigate and treat the people who are suffering from any abnormality. Testing should be financially viable, both for cost of screening and treatment which must be effective. The effectiveness of screening should be indicated by a reduction in the incidence of the condition after screening programmes are established.

The concept of screening for cervical cancer is based at present on an incompletely proven hypothesis of the aetiology and progress of the condition. The follow-up of women with signs of dysplasia representing various grades of cervical intraepithelial neoplasia (CIN) now suggests that in many early cases the condition resolves itself spontaneously. The more severe changes gradually progress, however, over 10–15 years or so to an invasive carcinoma which requires treatment. It is therefore possible that many women have the chance to complete their families long before surgical treatment becomes necessary. More rarely, the condition proceeds with haste and may be impossible to treat completely by the time the diagnosis is established. In a few cases the tumour may be hormone-dependent and may be activated by pregnancy or oral contraception.

There are no standard guidelines set out for the spacing between smears. Generally nurses working in family planning clinics will find that most women have a smear at or soon after their first clinic visit and thereafter at intervals of between one and five years. Where a smear has never been previously obtained or when there has been an exceptionally long interval it is usual for the laboratory to recommend a repeat in 12 months.

In some cases, because of infection, smears may be taken to isolate specific conditions of moniliasis and trichomoniasis. Occasionally mildly atypical smears may require repeating in just a few months. There is a wide diversity of opinion regarding the optimum spacing for cervical smears and nurses may find that it is helpful to discuss the spacing of routine smears with the doctors in the clinic where they work in order to be able to explain to the women the whys and wherefores of their recall periods. Questions commonly arise if it is discovered that friends and neighbours are receiving different recommendations. If the woman understands the reasons for the spacing applicable to her own case considerable anxiety can be avoided.

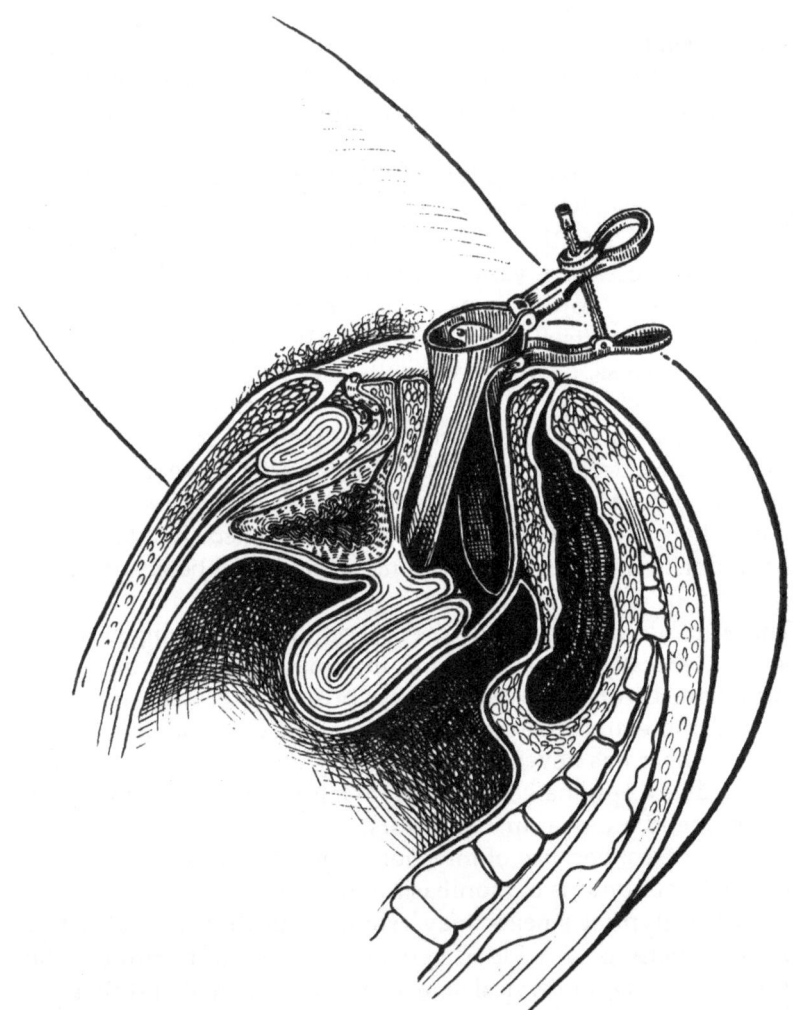

Figure 12.1 Insertion of cusco's speculum.

12.2 VAGINAL INSPECTION

In order to see the vagina clearly it is helpful to position the woman comfortably on her back with her legs abducted and to use good mobile illumination from an anglepoise lamp. The cervix protrudes about a centimetre into the anterior wall of the vagina and is seen by inserting a warm lubricated cusco's speculum downwards and backwards into the vagina and opening it gently when the cervix will come into view (Figure 12.1). The appearance and position of the cervix should be noted. When finally removing the speculum the jaws must be closed after withdrawing it a short distance or otherwise the cervix will become trapped in the blades. The technique requires some practice before confidence is established and careful supervision of beginners is essential. A woman who has not had a cervical smear taken within the last year needs one at booking or shortly afterwards. Women who resist vaginal examination, or repeatedly defer it, should be given every opportunity to discuss the reasons for their fears.

12.3 OBTAINING A CERVICAL SMEAR

While the cusco's speculum is in position for a vaginal inspection, the smear is obtained by passing a specially shaped spatula over the cervix with the shaped end resting in the cervical os. This should provide cells from the squamo-columnar junction (Figure 2.5, p. 14). Both wooden and plastic spatulae are available and various types are shown in Figure 12.2. The spatula is removed and should immediately have its collection thinly smeared on a glass slide which has already been marked on the frosted end in pencil with the woman's name, clinic number and date. The slide must not be allowed to dry out as this will damage the cells and make them difficult or even impossible to examine, and for this reason it is dipped immediately or sprayed with a thin film of fixative which is a mixture of ether and alcohol.

Taking a smear is not painful and is quickly and easily performed. Regular screening for cervical pre-cancer and cancer allows early diagnosis and treatment. It is however an expensive service and should be used selectively so that unnecessary duplication is not allowed to hinder rapid reporting. Women who are screened should be told that they are being tested only for cervical cancer, not endometrial or ovarian cancer, and it is

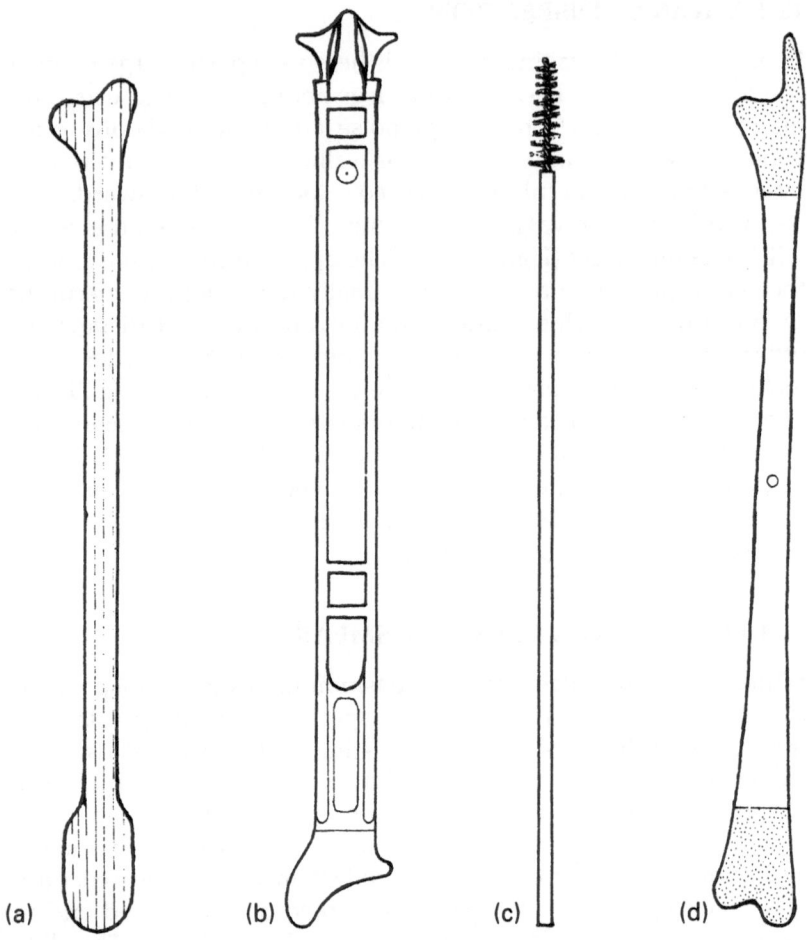

Figure 12.2 Spatulae for obtaining cervical cells, (a) wooden ayres; (b) aylsbury; (c) brush; (d) plastic ayres.

imperative that any irregular bleeding or other symptom must be reported to a doctor.

An important part of the nurse's contribution to a satisfactory service is to ensure that the cervical cytology form (Figure 12.3) is properly completed and accompanies the slide. Details of the woman's history will be in her records, but it is far easier just to ask the patient herself and this will get over the problems of the changed address or general practitioner.

HMR 101/5 (1982)

| 01 PATIENT'S HOSPITAL OR CLINIC CASE REFERENCE NO. | 10 NAME AND ADDRESS (TOWN) OF LABORATORY | 11 SLIDE SERIAL NO. |

02

SURNAME _____ MAIDEN NAME _____

FIRST NAMES _____

FULL POSTAL ADDRESS _____

03

IF HOSPITAL STATE:-

A

NAME AND ADDRESS OF SENDER IF NOT GP

CONSULTANT _____

WARD _____

HOSPITAL _____

Fold for B

| 04 DATE OF BIRTH | DAY | MONTH | YEAR | 05 NHS NO. |

Fold for A

06 SOURCE OF SMEAR	GP 1	HOSPITAL 4
	AHA 2	Other 5
	FP CLINIC 3	

07 HUSBAND'S OCCUPATION (patient's if unmarried) also state if Manager, Foreman or other

08

B

NAME AND ADDRESS OF GP

| 09 SPECIMEN TYPE | Cervical scrape 1 | Vaginal sample 2 | Cyto pipette 4 | Other (specify) 8 | LOCAL CODES | 26 27 28 29 30 |

Request/Report/Recall Form for Cervical or Vaginal Cytology – GP's COPY

| 12 MARITAL STATE | 13 PREGNANCES | 14 CONDITION | DATE OF | DAY | MTH | YR |

12 MARITAL STATE
Single 1
Married 2
Widowed/ 3
Divorced

13 PREGNANCES
Total births (live and still)
Total of abortions and miscarriages

14 CONDITION
Pregnant 1
Post-natal (under 12 weeks) 2
IUCD fitted 16
On oral contraceptive 4
On other hormones (specify in Box 21) 8

15 THIS TEST
16 LMP (1st day)
17 LAST TEST
18 NO PREVIOUS TEST (put x)

20 APPEARANCE OF CERVIX
Normal 1
Eroded 2
Cervicitis 4
Polyps 8
Malignant 16

19 SYMPTOMS
Discharge 1
Post-coital bleeding 2
Inter-menstrual bleeding 4
Post-menopausal bleeding 8
Other symptoms (Specify in Box 21) 16

21 CLINICAL DATA (PREVIOUS TREATMENT INCLUDING RADIO THERAPY/CHEMOTHERAPY)

22 CYTOLOGY REPORT

signature

Fold

23 EVIDENCE OF NEOPLASIA CYTOLOGICAL PATTERN SUGGESTS:
Inadequate specimen 1
Negative 2
Mild dysplasia 3
Severe dysplasia/ carcinoma-in-situ 4
Carcinoma-in-situ/? invasive 5
? Glandular neoplasia 6

24 INFLAMMATION
Severe Inflammatory Change 1
Trichomonas 2
Candida 4
Viral 8

25 FURTHER INVESTIGATION SUGGESTED
Repeat smear in ___ months 1
or after treatment 2
Colposcopy 16
Cervical biopsy 4
Uterine curettage 8

Signature _____   date _____

Fold

WRITE FIRMLY WITH BALLPOINT PEN ON A HARD SURFACE OR BACK COPY WILL BE ILLEGIBLE

ENTER DETAILS IN BOXES OR RING APPROPRIATE NUMBERS

Figure 12.3 Specimen of the report form for cervical cytology.

To accurately assess the normality of the cells on the slide the pathologist should know the age of the woman and whether the cervix appeared normal or inflamed. The appearance of the cells varies according to the alteration in strength of ovarian hormones, so the date of the last normal menstrual period is important and whether the patient is taking an oral contraceptive is significant. The woman's parity is recorded, as the proportion of columnar cells from the cervical canal will usually be greater in someone who has given birth owing to the stretched external cervical os. The presence of an intrauterine device may, similarly, alter the cellular pattern and should be recorded on the cervical cytology request form. Smears should not be taken during menstruation as the blood cells become attached to the slide and make inspection of the other cells difficult.

12.4 BIMANUAL PELVIC EXAMINATION

Nurses who have undertaken specialist training will be able to perform a complete examination of the pelvic organs. They must have a certificate of competence following specific clinical training, and even then continuing experience in the procedure is vital. The nurse's role is to establish whether the pelvic findings are normal and to refer out of the ordinary findings to a doctor for diagnosis.

Having taken the cervical smear, the speculum is carefully removed and the size of the introitus assessed. In sexually active women it will usually admit both the index and middle fingers: sometimes one has to make do with the index finger alone. The gloved fingers of the right hand are well lubricated with a water-based jelly; the labia are gently separated with the other hand and the examining fingers are slipped into the vagina in the same direction as the previous speculum insertion. Identify the cervix, feel that it is regular and smooth before sweeping the finger tips around the fornices. Now place the external hand on the lower abdomen and under gentle pressure the uterus can usually be felt between the two hands. The uterus should be mobile and movement should not cause discomfort in either lateral fornix. If the uterus is retroverted (Figure 12.4) it can be very difficult to identify, and pressure on the posterior surface of the uterine body through the posterior fornix causes discomfort. (A history of dyspareunia on deep penetration may accompany this finding.) The retroverted uterus may have been suspected by

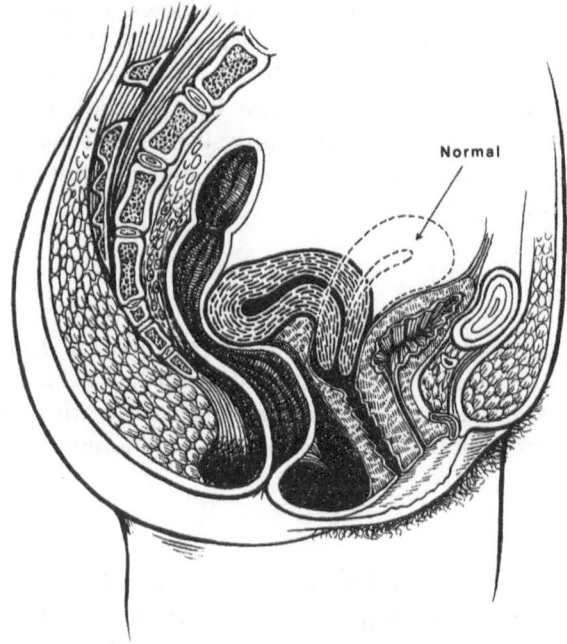

Figure 12.4 Retroverted uterus.

observing the angle of the cervix during speculum examination.

The normal ovary is not usually felt because of its size. However if it is enlarged it will be apparent in either lateral fornix when compressed between both hands. Other abnormalities of the adnexae include swollen fallopian tubes due to infection and, given the right history, an ectopic pregnancy.

This examination should also be undertaken when a coil-check is performed, as the stem of an IUD which has slipped into the cervical canal may not be seen on inspection, but can easily be felt as a hard rod in the external cervical os.

A clear record needs to be included in the woman's notes stating that a smear has been obtained and commenting on the cervical appearance and any abnormal discharge. Both normal and abnormal pelvic findings should be documented and signed.

12.5 RESULTS OF THE SMEAR

The patient will need to be informed of the result of her smear and simply suggesting that 'no news is good news' is not acceptable. Where it is impracticable to notify each patient and their GP the patient will need to make enquiry. In most cases nothing abnormal is detected. If, after staining by the Papinicolaou method, the cytology screening technician finds any suspicious cells, the slide is examined by the pathologist who will then write his assessment and recommendations.

Atypical cells

When infection is present atypical cells are apparent and a repeat smear needs to be taken when the infection has been treated. In some cases examination of the smear reveals a specific diagnosis of the type of infection such as moniliasis or trichomoniasis.

Dyskariosis

This name implies that an abnormal nucleus has developed, which may be the first indication of potential change within the cell towards over-activity. The changes in the nucleus are those of enlargement and irregularity of the boundary, due to an increase in chromatin content. In these cases a further smear is taken as soon as possible if the changes are severe, but it is quite possible to delay for a short while where the report is mild to moderate.

Cervical intra-epithelial neoplasia (CIN)

Whilst dyskariosis applies descriptively to shed cells present on a cervical smear, CIN refers to growing tissue present in the cervical epithelium. Where a biopsy is indicated the tissue which is removed will be examined and the cellular structure will either be reported as normal or given a CIN grading between 1 and 3. Sometimes on the cervical smear a guidance is given to the expected level of CIN involvement represented by the degree of dyskariosis observed.

Carcinoma *in situ*

This terminology has rather fallen into disuse and is more correctly represented by a grading of CIN 3.

Invasive carcinoma

This may be diagnosed only where there is histological evidence to show that the active cells are invading deeper tissue layers. Whilst it may be very suspicious from its appearance it is essential that confirmation is obtained from biopsy.

12.6 TREATMENT OF CIN

Markedly abnormal smears were treated previously by cone biopsy of the cervix where a cone-shaped piece of tissue was removed from the cervix to include affected ectocervix, the squamo-columnar junction and part of the endocervical canal. This approach to the problem was not without complication. More localized destruction of abnormal cells can now be achieved with the use of lasers, cool tissue coagulators and cryotherapy, which freezes any cells in contact with the special probe: all of these treatments can be painlessly effected and specifically directed at colposcopy in an appropriately equipped hospital out-patient department.

Colposcopy

This technique looks directly at the cells on the surface of the cervix using a specially mounted, low magnifying microscope. The patient needs to be placed in the lithotomy position and a speculum is positioned to disclose the cervix. The cervical surface is then painted with dilute acetic acid when the ectocervix and the cervical canal will reveal areas of cellular activity. Extra numbers of blood vessels and abnormal epithelial appearances also lead to suspicious areas becoming identified for selective biopsy, and these provide more accurate information for decisions about further treatment. Most colposcopy is carried out as an outpatient procedure, is usually painless and takes about half an hour.

13

Infection of the reproductive organs

While most women suffering from infection of the reproductive organs will lose no time in seeking help from their general practitioner, some will delay. The nurse working in family planning will find that a number of women will have anxieties, very often arising as a result of vaginal discharge. During routine visits, queries about infections should be dealt with promptly and the causative organism identified so that effective treatment can be given. An infection may be discovered only as a result of following up anxieties voiced by the woman during her visit to the clinic. Occasionally the nurse will notice that the vaginal discharge has an unpleasant odour; if so, she should tactfully enquire about this and mention it to the doctor.

All nurses working in family planning clinics should be familiar with the common types of vaginal infection and causes of discharge which are discussed in this chapter. It will enable them to recognize and offer appropriate advice to women who are frequently very self-conscious and distressed about the symptoms, and who may not always have the courage to speak to the doctor without encouragement and support. In certain cases it may be preferable for an infection to be treated in a clinic dealing with genito–urinary disorders (or 'special clinic') where facilities for diagnosis and contact tracing are more effective. Infections dealt with in special clinics are not necessarily sexually transmitted, and this should be explained before the woman is referred. Most district general hospitals have a genito–urinary clinic, a complete list of which may be obtained from the local Health Education Council, District Health Authority's offices or a general practitioner's surgery.

13.1 VAGINAL THRUSH
(CANDIDIASIS OR VAGINAL MONILIASIS)

This fungal infection of the vagina is very common. The fungus is present (but often dormant) in a quarter of the female population of childbearing age. In about 30% of this group the fungus multiplies and produces symptoms of vulval and vaginal irritation with a characteristic odour and a white cheesy discharge seen on the vaginal epithelium and cervix. The remaining 70% are unaware of the condition so long as the acidity of the vagina is maintained. This acidity is provided by the Döderlein's bacilli which are naturally present there, making use of the glycogen formed in the vaginal cells and the cervical mucus. If the Döderlein's bacilli are destroyed, for example by a course of antibiotic, or if excess vaginal exudate dilutes the acidity as in pregnancy, then the fungal development which has previously been inhibited by the acid pH starts to proliferate and cause irritation. The use of oral contraceptives similarly may provoke these symptoms. Likewise, during the menopause intermittent thrush may develop as the acidity of the vagina becomes less strong when the lining cells provide less nourishment for the Döderlein's bacilli. Diabetics have a higher incidence of moniliasis because there is less glycogen in the vaginal cells, and there is the possibility of contamination of the area with glycosuria.

Moniliasis is not peculiar to sexually active women, but whilst visiting a contraceptive clinic women may feel able to speak about the problem more freely than with their family doctor. There may be facilities for making a firm diagnosis, and vaginal examination is far easier in the clinic environment. Delay in seeking advice may result in severe irritation and later oedema which is so bad as to cause pain, dyspareunia and insomnia. Advice should always cover both partners and it is helpful if the man can be encouraged to use an anti-fungal cream to prevent the harbouring of any spores underneath his foreskin ready to cause reinfection. While the treatment is taking place it is quite helpful for intercourse to continue, if this is possible without too much discomfort, so that both partners receive treatment from the anti-monilial substance inserted into the vagina. This treatment may be in the form of cream or pessaries.

Definitive diagnosis can be made on speculum examination in most cases except where severe oedema and inflammation makes the procedure far too painful. Yeasts can be identified, preferably from a scraping of the lateral vaginal wall or from a high vaginal swab (HVS) and may need to be cultured if no organisms are identified on direct microscopy. Often the cervical smear is helpful and shows spores and hyphae which are the chains of growing fungal cells.

Modern treatment of monilia is effective, providing that adequate levels of medication are achieved and foci of reinfection from the ever-present bowel spores are eliminated. Until recently nystatin in the form of cream and pessaries was singularly satisfactory, but newer substances such as miconazole, econazole and clotrimazole have become available and they are strikingly effective in most cases. Pessaries can be inserted at night high up in the vagina or creams may be similarly positioned with the use of an applicator. This is a simple syringe which is filled from the tube and an additional small application is rubbed into the skin of the vulva to abolish local irritation.

Systemic treatment may sometimes be necessary where the infection is difficult to clear, and ketoconazole 200–400 mg is effective by mouth providing there are no contraindications. Oral nystatin (which is not absorbed from the gut) 500 000 units taken six hourly will prevent a potential source of reinfection from the lower bowel. If there is extreme discomfort and oedema it may be necessary to arrange a short hospital admission and treatment of the condition by vulval toilet and painting with aqueous gentian violet. This is less often required nowadays, but can be very effective and soothing. Unfortunately it is messy, staining linen and underclothes; but this may be kept to a minimum with careful application and suitable protection.

If the woman has recently had a baby, or is pregnant, she should be warned about the risk of cross-infection to young children, and the basic elements of personal hygiene, hand washing, food and milk preparation should be clearly explained. It may also be wise to describe the symptoms of oral thrush in babies so that she can identify it should it occur and quickly obtain treatment.

Women who are treated for infection should avoid nylon pants, using cotton instead, and avoid the use of panti-hose tights and close fitting jeans and trousers which may cause abrasions and prevent reasonable ventilation. The use of vaginal deodorants and strongly scented bath preparations may be responsible for allergic responses and infection may be encouraged by the alteration of the normal vaginal acidity and flora. A solution of household vinegar 1:20 with tap water poured over an inflamed vulva will provide rapid relief as a first-aid measure.

13.2 *TRICHOMONAS VAGINALIS*

This parasitic infection is found in both men and women and probably affects at least 20% of women at some time during their childbearing years. It is most commonly transferred during sexual intercourse and is rarely to be found in women before they become sexually active.

Trichomonas vaginalis is a unicellular motile organism which is propelled by its flagellae, which are situated at one end. It inhabits the deep folds of the lining of the vagina and may very well be asymptomatic for long periods of time. A change in vaginal acidity may cause a proliferation of the parasite, which is then responsible for infection of the surrounding tissues, causing swelling and a frothy green and occasionally bloodstained discharge with an unpleasant odour. The infection may also be found in the lower urethra and the associated Skene's glands, and can be responsible for infecting Bartholin's glands. The incubation period following infection at intercourse is 7–21 days. In severe cases there is considerable pain and swelling and there may be pain on micturition. The partner is usually asymptomatic, but sometimes discharge and dysuria may be present.

The diagnosis can be made by observing under the microscope a sample of the discharge diluted with isotonic saline, when the parasite can be seen moving about using its flagellae. If the parasite cannot be seen or there is no microscope available a high vaginal swab of the discharge should be sent in transport medium to the laboratory for culture. Samples may also be fixed on a slide similarly to cervical cytology.

Treating the couple with oral metronidazole (Flagyl) should be effective and 200 mg are taken three times a day for seven days. It should be stressed that both partners must receive treatment. Where there appears to be doubt about the likelihood of regular tablet taking it is possible to give the metronidazole as three 1 g doses at twelve-hourly intervals; however with this higher dose there is an increased risk of side effects. A warning should be given that alcohol is better avoided whilst under treatment with metronidazole for it may speed up the excretion of the drug, reducing the quantity in tissues so that it is not as effective. It also has an emetic effect similar to disulfiram (Antabuse) which is a drug used in the treatment of alcoholism.

It is always advisable for a repeat smear to be taken six weeks after treatment. Ideally, the woman should be rechecked in three months to ensure treatment has been successful. At this stage a few cases will require a further course of medication. It is not uncommon to find that women suffering from trichomoniasis also have gonorrhoea, so tests for this possibility must be considered.

13.3 *GARDNERELLA VAGINALIS*

This common organism causes an offensive smelling vaginal discharge but without any irritation as it is not a tissue pathogen and does not produce any inflammatory response. The possibility of it co-existing with other vaginal infections must be borne in mind. In the majority of cases treatment with metronidazole is completely effective.

13.4 CHLAMYDIA

This is one of the commonest sexually transmitted diseases. It is caused by the presence of chlamydial organisms which give rise to a vaginal discharge which is non-irritant, and of varying amount. Once the infection becomes established it affects the upper genital tract so that left untreated it becomes a common cause of salpingitis and all the inherent complications. The organism may contaminate a neonate during its passage through the birth canal causing opthalmic discharge.

This organism is identified from a swab passed right into the endocervix and rotated so that it collects endocervical cells. The specimen may be specially cultured although the organism is most easily recognized by rolling the culture swab over a special glass microscope slide, which is dispatched to a laboratory where it is examined by dark ground immunofluorescence.

Treatment is oxytetracycline or its derivative doxycycline but where there is contraindication, erythromycin may be used just as effectively. Oxytetracycline and erythromycin are given by mouth in a dosage of 250 mg four times a day for 14 days, whereas doxycycline is effective after a loading dose of 200 mg followed by 100 mg three times daily for the same period.

13.5 GONORRHOEA

The gonococcus is a germ with a long history. The disease has been recognized since ancient times and is thought to have been referred to in several biblical texts; for instance when Moses had all the potentially infected Midianite women slaughtered! (Numbers 31, 14–18). Certainly an effective remedy but perhaps a little drastic by today's standards! It is still a highly infectious disease and is the third most common notifiable disease in the UK, only beaten in the statistics by measles and non-specific genital infection.

The condition is spread by infected persons during intercourse, and has an incubation period of 2–10 days. This may extend to a period of several weeks in women who remain asymptomatic and the infection may only be discovered by contact tracing. The gonococcus lodges in the urethra, Bartholin's glands, endocervical canal and sometimes the rectum. It does not survive in an adult vagina because it cannot penetrate the normal keratinized skin, but young children can suffer from vaginal infection as a result of poor hygiene in a household where an adult is affected. The gonococcus is very susceptible to changes in temperature and only survives in a moist warm atmosphere. This point is important when culture of the organism is necessary. Swabs need to be immediately dispatched to the laboratory which has to be able to handle them without delay if infections are not to go undiagnosed.

The women who suffer symptoms may develop a Bartholin's abscess. Infection of the urethra may cause some mild discomfort on micturition. Perhaps the commonest symptom is a mild non-irritant vaginal discharge which originates from the cervix. From the cervix the infection spreads into the uterus and along the fallopian tubes with symptoms of lower abdominal pain, *malaise* and pyrexia. The resulting salpingitis causes stenosis of the tubes and may give rise to complete sterility: occasionally a pelvic abscess may develop creating retort shaped tubes and peritonitis follows. Infection of the rectum also occurs even in the absence of practising anal intercourse as the infection can spread from the perineum to the rectum and cause proctitis.

In men the symptoms generally appear 3–5 days following the initial infection and include discomfort on micturition and purulent discharge from the urethral meatus. If treatment is delayed or ignored the infection can spread to the epididymis with scrotal swelling and associated pain which can extend into the perineum.

Left untreated, permanent damage can occur and a urethral stricture may develop causing great difficulty with micturition.

Diagnosis

If a smear of urethral discharge is stained by Gram's method and examined microscopically under ordinary illumination the gonococci show up as paired, intracellular, bean shaped diplococci. False negatives can easily occur unless care is taken with the culture material. A scrape from the urethral canal with a platinum loop will provide pus cells containing the organism. Final diagnosis requires even more care as between 10 and 30% of cases can be missed. The urethral smears should be taken and sent, without delay, to the laboratory along with cervical and rectal smears transported in Stuart's medium. In special clinics the organisms are inoculated onto a culture dish and covered with a candle jar to minimize delays.

Treatment

It is vital that the woman and partner are treated, and a service of contact tracing has been established in the special clinics to enable all contacts to be traced confidentially and offered treatment. Penicillin in a variety of combinations is used, and where the gonococcus shows resistance the dose needs to be increased. It is important that the blood level of penicillin is raised throughout the 24 hours in order to be effective. Usually 2–3 g ampicillin are given at once by mouth along with 1 g probenecid, which delays the excretion of penicillin through the kidneys. Alternatively 5 Mega U of benzyl penicillin are given by intramuscular injection with 5 ml of 0.5% lignocaine added to relieve the pain and discomfort of injecting so large a volume. Oral probenecid is given at the same time. Other effective preparations are available for those individuals allergic to penicillin and its derivatives. Follow up tests are usually performed 4–7 days after treatment to confirm success, and during that time both partners should avoid alcohol. Neither partner should resume sexual activity until tests prove the treatment has been successful.

It is essential that each clinic follows a routine of impeccable cleanliness in its management of equipment, couches, dressing gowns, changing rooms and disposal of rubbish: particular care is needed when an infected person has been seen. Gloves should always be worn when cleaning and washing equipment. When the clinics are held in old buildings, or the number of people is larger than usual, or there is a shortage of staff, it becomes difficult to maintain standards. Fatigue sets in and there is greater risk of cross-infection. In these circumstances extra effort has to be made by all staff to maintain a really high standard of cleanliness throughout the clinic.

13.6 SYPHILIS

This disease is considerably rarer than gonorrhoea, although the two are often found together. The infection is caused by the organism *Treponema pallidum*, which may be identified in the lesions and later appears systemically in the blood and all body tissues. The incubation period for this disease is 9–90 days, but it most commonly occurs 3–4 weeks after intercourse with an infected partner. An ulcer, otherwise known as a primary chancre, is found on or near the external sex organs. This ulcer is painless but highly infectious and gradually heals over the course of the next few weeks. The adjacent inguinal lymph glands often become swollen. In women the ulcer is usually found on one or other labia, or it may appear on the cervix. The lesion may be quite uncharacteristic and any ulcer occurring in this area must at least be considered as possibly representing syphilis, in view of the early spontaneous healing which does not advertise the more dangerous generalized infection which is continuing to affect the whole body.

So far we have dealt with only the primary infection, but if the disease remains undiagnosed and untreated, further symptoms such as fever, sore throat and skin rashes appear a few weeks later. Once again, these effects disappear without any treatment. The disease however remains in the body and if still untreated can result in symptoms closely resembling many other diseases. Its late tertiary effects on the central nervous system cause paralysis and mental deterioration.

Diagnosis

Various blood tests are available for the diagnosis of syphilis. A general screening for this is done by using two tests: the Reagin test and the Venereal Disease Reference Laboratory test (VDRL). Both show a small margin of error and used together they eliminate most of the false positives and negatives which can occur when only one is used. A more specific test, the Treponemal Haemaglutination Assessment (TPHA) is carried out if the other tests are positive. Where there is doubt about the diagnosis the Fluorescent Treponemal Antibody test (FTA) may be used. The more specific tests have the inconvenience of needing special laboratory facilities. In the past the Wasserman (WR) test was used but it was non-specific and had a wide margin of error, giving positive results for a number of other conditions including yaws and lymphogranuloma venereum, so that it is hardly, if ever, used nowadays. Direct smears from infected sites can be examined under a microscope using the technique of dark ground illumination. This enables immediate diagnosis to be made and speedy treatment given.

Treatment

As with gonorrhoea, treatment needs to be prompt and effective and is best given in a specialist department where accurate diagnosis can be made. Penicillin is still effective and intramuscular injections of procaine penicillin are best. Sometimes erythromycin is given orally. Good contact tracing is important in controlling the disease and allows for earlier treatment where it is found to be necessary. The indiscriminate and inadequate use of antibiotics results in masking the disease which then remains dormant to become dangerously active many years later. The primary chancre is still the best known symptom and is the best time to deal with the infection.

13.7 ACQUIRED IMMUNE DEFICIENCY SYNDROME (AIDS)

Considerable concern is being expressed about this viral disease. Human immunosuppressive virus (HIV, previously described as HTLV) is primarily transferred from an infected person by sexual intercourse or by contamination with infected blood. The virus reproduces in the T lymphocytes and interferes with the body's ability to control infection. There is a variable latent phase between the initial infection and collapse of the defence system and serious illness which is likely to be terminal. An asymptomatic carrier state can exist.

An intensive programme to control this epidemic is being undertaken by all western governments until an effective treatment is found. The use of condoms, preferably with impregnated spermicide, is strongly advised and avoidance of casual intercourse will reduce the risk of infection and dispersion. The recent discovery that benzylkonium chloride (nonoxynol 9, 10 & 11), used in some countries as a spermicide, effectively kills the virus on contact is encouraging news. Owing to the rapidly increasing incidence of this disease and the associated publicity it is likely that many health professionals are going to come into contact with people who have anxieties. These must be dealt with in an informed and sympathetic way and if the client requests tests to confirm absence of the virus it is essential that they are referred to an AIDS counsellor.

One of the outcomes of this outbreak has been to stress the importance of the need for health professionals to be meticulous in avoidance of cross-infection by their observation of hygiene and cleanliness. In the event of a health worker sustaining damage by potentially contaminated needles or sharp instruments it is advisable to encourage bleeding from the site of injury, to wash the site well with any disinfectant solution and to seek immediate medical advice.

13.8 GENITAL HERPES

Genital herpes is caused by the herpes simplex type II virus (type I is generally an oral pathogen). It is reasonably common and is sometimes found in association with other venereal diseases. The ulcers, unlike those of syphilis, are painful and multiple and are associated in the first instance with blister formation and swelling of the inguinal lymph glands. The characteristic herpetic lesions in the female are found most commonly on the vulva, from which they are inclined to spread onto the perineum and the upper thighs. There is usually local irritation to start with and then single or multiple vesicles follow. Herpes is commonly found on the cervix and the disease appears to have a high correlation with cervical pre-cancer and possibly cancer. Nursing staff should be on the alert for this and make sure that these women have regular annual smears. In the male the herpetic vesicles may be found on glands, under the prepuce and less frequently on the shaft of the penis. Very rarely the scrotum itself may be involved. As well as being painful this condition has the troublesome habit of recurring.

Diagnosis

The diagnosis may be confirmed by taking a smear in the same way as for cervical exfoliative cytology, fixed ready for transport to the laboratory. Virology studies may be available in some laboratories and material should be sent in virus transport medium. Certain antibodies to the two existing herpes simplex viruses can be determined in blood but are not specific for type and are only of limited value.

Treatment

Treatment is difficult, but worth attempting in order to try and relieve symptoms which are particularly distressing as the disease has the tendency to recur in susceptible individuals. It may be possible to paint some of the external lesions with 5% idoxuridine but this will, at best, have only a limited effect. Acyclovir, which is also an anti-viral agent, has a place in controlling the acute herpetic symptoms if taken early enough, but has not achieved the hope of a long-term cure.

13.9 GENITAL WARTS

These are known as condylomata accuminata. There has been a great increase in the incidence of this disease and perhaps it is a reflection of the increased sexual freedom which has occurred since the contraceptive pill has been available. The incubation period is a long one: several months may elapse before the warts appear, which makes contact tracing extremely difficult to carry out where there is more than a single partner. The warts initially appear in females on the vulva or perineum and may spread up the vagina and cover the cervix. In the male the lesion is usually found on the frenum but later other warts may be found on the shaft of the penis. Because of their viral nature warts may seed themselves in adjacent sites so that a lesion on one side of the vulva rapidly spreads to the other side or across the perineum.

Treatment

In the female the affected part is painted with podophylline paint to prevent mitosis (cell division). The outer parts of the vulva and perineum are painted with either a 10 or 25% solution of podophylline in Tinct. Benz. Co., whilst the inner aspect of the labia and introitus are painted with the lower strength solution of podophylline only. In males the penis is treated in the same manner. Only the immediately affected area is painted and it is important to be sure that it is dry before the individual replaces their clothing. Instruction is given about taking a bath eight hours afterwards to wash off any remaining paint. Depending on the extent of the disease the painting is carried out either every other day or weekly, and if there is no benefit then more radical treatment is necessary with cautery, diathermy or freezing of the individual warts. Sometimes surgical excision is required.

Like the common skin wart, genital warts may regress spontaneously and indeed many of the satisfactory results may simply depend on time. Anyone who has genital warts must be considered a potential candidate for other venereal diseases. In males the commonest of these is non-specific urethritis; in women it is candidiasis; and one may expect more rapid elimination of the warts when these infections have been effectively treated.

13.10 GENITAL INFESTATIONS

Less commonly encountered, infestations of scabies and pubic lice may be diagnosed. These are dealt with by the use of benzyl benzoate scrub or gamma benzene hexachloride respectively.

13.11 BACTEROIDES SPECIES

These are bowel organisms which are likely to cause pelvic infection in females. Until recently they went unrecognized, but they have probably been at the seat of many long term cases of chronic pelvic sepsis in the past. Treatment is now quite easily effected with the standard dose of metronidazole either in the form of tablets or vaginal pessaries.

13.12 BETA HAEMOLYTIC STREPTOCOCCUS

This organism appears to be taking an increasing responsibility for causing vaginal discharge. It usually responds to treatment with one of the penicillins or more up-to-date derivatives.

13.13 ATROPHIC VAGINITIS

Diminishing levels of oestrogen following the menopause or after bilateral oophorectomy may be the cause of vaginal dryness and discomfort. The symptoms may be noticed at any time but are often more pronounced with intercourse. Cells forming the vaginal wall become fragile when they do not receive enough oestrogen and the inadequate lining is prone to damage and infection. A history may also be given of brown discharge or even bleeding, and what may turn out to be a difficult vaginal examination reveals areas of excoriation.

Local application of oestrogen cream provides rapid improvement in symptoms but care must be taken that this is only used with correct medical supervision. Post-menopausal bleeding is always cause for a gynaecological opinion. In some instances it may be appropriate to use oral oestrogen or subcutaneous implant therapy. There has been a recent development of small adhesive patches containing oestrogen which gets absorbed through the skin; the patches are replaced twice weekly and look as if they are going to be most useful in treating all menopausal symptoms.

13.14 FOREIGN BODIES

Sometimes women are concerned about particularly offensive vaginal discharge which will turn out to be due to a foreign body in the vagina. The commonest of these is a tampon, but may occasionally be a lost condom. The main symptom of the presence of foreign bodies is that the discharge is more than usually offensive and malodorous. It is not restricted to people with low intelligence: nobody is immune, but it is always a source of much embarrassment and necessitates particular understanding. The removal of the offending article is usually sufficient to bring an end to the distressing symptoms and only occasionally is a broad spectrum antibiotic necessary if the vaginal mucosa is damaged.

13.15 RETAINED PRODUCTS OF CONCEPTION

This condition may produce varying amounts of bloodstained vaginal discharge. The colour will be bright red if a fresh event but if older it will appear brown. Whilst it may follow childbirth it is as likely to be associated with spontaneous miscarriage or termination of pregnancy. The history will usually reveal whether the abortion was complete or not and in some cases an early pregnancy may have ceased to grow, died and been retained in the uterus (missed abortion). The woman must be seen and examined by a doctor who will probably discover on vaginal examination that the cervix is open and refer her to hospital for further investigation such as ultrasound scanning and where necessary a dilatation and currettage (D & C).

13.16 URINARY TRACT INFECTION

Although this is not an infection of the reproductive organs it is a common complaint in contraceptive clinics and is therefore included to complete the chapter. In most cases the woman complains of cystitis and will have experienced the symptoms previously. If the infection is promptly and adequately dealt with it should not recur; unfortunately some people can suffer from it intermittently over many years. The symptoms of dysuria and frequency of micturition with or without haematuria should be reported to the doctor. A midstream specimen of urine should be sent to the laboratory for culture and sensitivity.

Collecting a midstream specimen of urine

In order to obtain a midstream specimen of urine, the woman should be clearly instructed to wash her labia majora and minora with clean water and dry herself with the sterile wool swabs provided. The urine should be passed into the lavatory and a sterile kidney dish inserted between the legs during voiding to catch a sample. There are some good disposable kits on the market which are pre-sterilized and provide a plastic funnel to direct the urine specimen into the container, and these avoid the use of a separate kidney dish and reduce the risk of contaminating the sample. The woman should be discouraged from stopping and starting the stream as this is not only difficult but defeats the object of midstream clarity. Rather, the collecting device should pass into the flowing stream and be removed when sufficient sample has been collected. The task of explaining the above to women who do not speak English may be overcome by using an old teapot to demonstrate how to catch a midstream specimen!

Treatment

Treatment is usually commenced at once with one of the broad spectrum antibiotics which can be changed if the results of the MSU show a specific resistance. The nurse should take time to explain the nature of the antibiotic therapy, and emphasize the need to take the tablets regularly and finish the course completely so that resistance does not occur. The urine should be re-examined a week after the treatment is completed to make sure that it has been effective.

Some women have bacteruria which is asymptomatic, but is a potential problem as it is a reservoir of infection which can flare up. Chronic kidney infection known as pyelonephritis is a common and debilitating problem for many women in later life and may cause considerable distress and poor health. Some of these people can be spared this unfortunate prospect if minor urinary infections are effectively treated when they are younger.

Urinary infection following intercourse or 'honeymoon cystitis' occurs because the short female urethra is massaged during intercourse, encouraging bacteria to move up into the bladder. Advice on voiding urine shortly after intercourse can reduce the problem.

14

Special needs

14.1 NEEDS OF YOUNG PEOPLE

The number of young people who are in danger of becoming pregnant is high. Recent work on estimating the number of girls having intercourse before they were aged 16 gave a figure 1 in 8 (boys admitted, or boasted, 1 in 3) and many were exposed to possible pregnancy on several occasions before seeking contraceptive advice. Attitudes vary about young people having free access to contraception, and health professionals are often in personal conflict when approached by the young as to whether they should be involved in providing contraception for those below 16 years, the legal age of consent. The House of Lords has considered it to be lawful for a doctor to provide contraceptive services to a girl under 16 years of age providing it is in her best interest. It is perhaps timely to warn these young girls that their partners, whatever their own age, could be liable to prosecution for unlawful sexual intercourse because of their being below the age of consent.

On account of their nervousness some young people can behave badly at the first visit and this may not exactly endear them to the receptionist or other staff: it could get them off to a bad start if the personnel are not quick to recognize the need for reassurance. It requires considerable courage to enter a clinic for contraception and when the girl is young she will feel extremely apprehensive. Youth advisory clinics are staffed with sympathetic and experienced health personnel who know about the special needs of these young people. Too often girls delay coming until they are seriously worried about possible pregnancy or infection, and this will raise their anxiety levels further, so that friendly and receptive staff will be the most help.

The younger girl may come to the clinic or surgery with a friend as support and both should be made welcome. Occasionally the girl is brought by a parent, although this is unusual. Some parents are concerned and supportive, but a few are overbearing and try to make all the decisions which leads to difficulties. Whilst they must, of course, be included in the discussion, a delicate balance needs to be maintained and it is essential that the girl is given the opportunity of private discussion with the doctor or nurse to express her own views about the available methods and also to enlarge on any problems which she may not wish to talk about in her parent's presence. If an opportunity is not given for private discussion an early pregnancy or infection may be missed and the girl will never feel entirely sure that she can rely on the confidentiality of the staff. The fact that they are requesting a method of contraception must indicate a responsible attitude to the challenge of becoming an adult.

At the first visit a full history is required, but a medical examination may not necessarily be carried out; indeed it is better to wait until the girl has gained confidence and gets to know the clinic staff better. An exception will be necessary when there is the possibility of pregnancy or an infection which will require immediate investigation. Many young girls are understandably terrified of having vaginal examinations and if they have a bad experience they will be frightened to come back and may also deter their friends from seeking help.

A little time spent on discussing any previous efforts made to avoid pregnancy – and the method of contraception requested – will reveal which of the available methods is going to be the correct choice. It is extremely unlikely that any method will be consistently used as younger people are generally more erratic in their sexual behaviour.

Barrier methods require definitive motivation and forethought, and carrying sheaths may not be acceptable as it suggests that the girl is anticipating intercourse, which will place her in a difficult social predicament. Some young men will be motivated to carry sheaths and will use them successfully, but any lack of confidence over their ability to maintain an erection may be the basis of refusal to use this method. However, publicity over the AIDS crisis has provided the opportunity for further health education and encouragement for the use of a protective method which has improved the sheath's image and acceptability. Oral contraception would seem the most acceptable method, but although it has a high safety record this is dependent on regular use and of course it provides no protection against infection. Most doctors hesitate to put young girls on oral contraception until the menstrual cycle is fully established. However it may be justified if the girl is unhappy about using other methods and faces termination of pregnancy which is a much more dangerous and unsatisfactory alternative.

IUDs are not often used in young people. If the girl's partner is using withdrawal as a means of preventing conception the girl should be instructed in how to use this particular method and its limitations should be explained to her. The safe period is difficult to calculate in the early years as the cycle can be irregular and in any case this method does not fit with the lifestyle of impetuous youth. In clinics and surgeries staff should be conversant with post-coital contraception and make sure this service is available.

Abortion cannot be considered as a method of contraception and any young girl depending on it should be given time for full discussion on the wider implications of this operation and its effects on her future reproduction. This is a sad and difficult area of management. A number of young people find a decision on abortion difficult, and the girl must decide for herself without the influence of parents or boyfriend. If an operation is necessary one of her parents will have to know about the termination if she is under age and the girl will require considerable courage to face this situation. Despite disappointment, however, many parents will turn up trumps; a few may require some help to do so and this is where support and counselling may be helpful.

For those who find adjusting to sexual maturity difficult, sympathetic support given by health professionals is encouraging and may be all that is required. People attending a family planning clinic quite often have anxieties which they may find the courage to discuss with professional staff who handle them with attentive concern. If the nurse does not succeed in establishing a caring relationship with people she will not be approached and may therefore remain ignorant of their distress.

14.2 POSTPARTUM WOMEN

Women who have recently delivered a baby either in hospital or at home usually welcome an opportunity to discuss contraception with a midwife or health visitor. The couple may be perfectly satisfied with their previous contraceptive method which should not be altered if it met all their needs. The physiological changes after childbearing need to be discussed with the couple as these have implications in the use of all methods.

Postpartum physiology

During pregnancy a great deal of tissue growth occurs within the uterus and there is also a considerable increase in its vascularity. After delivery the uterus returns to its pre-pregnancy dimensions by a process of involution. Involution will at first be rapid and the uterus will reduce in size dramatically during the initial ten days. The unwanted tissue is broken down, digested, absorbed and excreted. After six weeks the uterus is usually back to its pre-pregnant size, and during this period the uterine wall is more friable than usual and more easily damaged, whilst the raw lining is susceptible to infection.

The increased levels of oestrogen and progesterone in the body during pregnancy decrease during the postpartum period but their effect takes time to wear off. The progesterone, which softens smooth muscle and allows for some give in the pelvic ligaments, may continue to influence muscle tone in the body for several weeks. This laxity is of particular significance in the vagina which has been stretched to accommodate the baby and varies in the speed with which it returns to normal. For this reason any attempt to fit a diaphragm cap in the postpartum period will be less accurate and require earlier re-assessment. Some perineal damage may have occurred with delivery and this usually heals well in two or three weeks. Occasionally problems with poor healing, haematoma or infection may prolong the discomfort.

Lactation

When successful breast feeding is established, lactation may continue for a year or more and during this time the return of menstruation and ovarian function may be delayed to some extent. The old wives' tale of not being able to conceive during lactation persists but unfortunately breast feeding cannot be relied upon as a contraceptive method. Many unplanned pregnancies have occurred in this way and mothers should be specifically warned about the risk. Work done by Dr Alan McNeilly and Professor Peter Howie at the MRC Unit of Reproductive Biology in Edinburgh on the action of breast feeding on ovarian function suggests that the key to successful suppression lies in good frequent stimulation of the nipple by demand feeding. This sets off a series of mechanisms which produce consistently high levels of prolactin in the blood and suppress gonadotrophin which in turn prevents ovulation. It is not known whether it is the prolactin or the afferent impulses to the hypothalamus which suppresses the ovulation. Unfortunately it is necessary for the baby to feed and stimulate the nipple regularly throughout the whole 24 hour period to maximize the contraceptive effect. The mother sleeping with her baby beside her and allowing frequent suckling day and night may be better protected, and this pattern of breast feeding is of great importance in reducing the number of births in those societies where no other form of birth control is used. If, as is common in our present society, the baby is encouraged to miss a night feed then the strength of the suckling stimulus will drop and ovulation may recur. As soon as the baby is weaned or given additional milk the prolactin level will fall and such a fall is commonly followed by ovulation evidenced by a period two weeks later. This ovulation being unheralded makes unprotected intercourse risky in the early weeks. Absence of menstruation is therefore no guarantee of contraceptive security.

The blood loss from the uterus known as lochia reduces quite rapidly within the first ten days becoming slight and odourless. In the absence of breast feeding the first period following delivery appears after six weeks: with established lactation it may not appear for many months.

Pregnancy occurring in the older age group has a higher incidence of morbidity and mortality for both mother and infant, so although it is less likely to occur an unplanned pregnancy near the menopause must be managed very carefully. Early ante-natal booking and screening with consultant supervision should be arranged.

Postnatal contraception

Mother and baby are safer, healthier and happier if there is an opportunity between pregnancies for the child to become well established and the mother to regain her physical and emotional stability. The WHO report quoting from international research suggests that siblings delivered within 18 months are often lighter in weight and less intelligent because of depleted maternal circumstances. The months after the arrival of a baby are exhausting and stressful for parents, and fear of another pregnancy may increase tension and make the relationship guarded and insular. Both parents need each other's love and affection at this time, whether or not they wish to recommence intercourse. An understanding midwife or health visitor who is able to recognize signs of stress will often pick these up and friendly discussion with both parents may help and encourage the couple to understand each other's needs.

The particular advantages and disadvantages of the various contraceptive methods for women in the first few weeks after childbirth are as follows.

Barrier methods

The best choice of the barrier methods is the sheath if the partner is prepared to use one for the first few weeks. Otherwise caps may be effectively fitted but they need constant supervision and frequent refitting at first. Recently healed perineal scar tissue may be sensitive. If the delivery was by caesarean section the cap can be fitted more easily and may well be satisfactory. Each woman needs to be assessed separately by the family planning nurse to ascertain who would be happier to use sheaths and who would be better suited to the cap.

Combined oral contraception

If this method has been used previously and the mother is not breast feeding she can recommence the pills at a convenient time within two weeks of delivery. Breast feeding mothers are advised not to use combined oral contraception until after weaning because the effect of the oestrogen is inclined to reduce lactation. This method may need to be reviewed if there have been any hypertensive episodes during pregnancy or if there has been any indication of gestational diabetes.

Progesterone-only pill

Whether or not the mother has used it before, this pill is ideal if she is breast feeding. It can be commenced at any time after the first 48 hours have elapsed or within two weeks following delivery. Whilst its effectiveness is slightly less than that of the combined pill it is probably enhanced by the raised level of prolactin and in no way diminishes the amount of milk produced. There is no adverse effect of progesterone on the breast-fed baby.

IUDs

In certain circumstances where the risk of pregnancy is great and other methods of contraception are not acceptable the mother may request an IUD. If a device is to be inserted into a recently pregnant uterus it should be done by an expert family planning doctor as the risk of perforation is higher, as is the chance of infection within the uterus which is still healing in the area of the placental site. As the uterine muscle contracts and retracts during the process of involution the size of the cavity will also reduce. If an IUD is inserted before six weeks post-delivery it is easily dislodged and extruded through the imperfectly reformed cervix. If this occurs the woman will not be protected against pregnancy and may also lose confidence in the method. On occasion an individual woman will request an early fitting and it may well turn out satisfactorily, but the nurse will need to make arrangements for her to be followed up more closely until the uterus is back to normal. If the device is too large when the uterus returns to normal it may become distorted and provide less efficient protection and be more difficult to remove subsequently. The optimum time to insert a postpartum IUD is at the postnatal examination about six weeks following delivery.

Postpartum sterilization

Although it would seem to be a convenient time for this relatively minor surgery to be carried out, it is far better for sterilization to be delayed until several weeks have elapsed since the baby's birth. Postoperative risks to the mother following early surgery are unacceptably high, and include haemorrhage and thrombosis which already provide postnatal hazard. Furthermore, the full implication of a permanent method of birth control needs careful reappraisal at a time when both parents can make a rational decision. It is also important that the new baby has time to establish itself and can be seen to be developing normally.

14.3 THE MENOPAUSE

The menopause describes the natural cessation of menstruation associated with the ending of ovarian function. This usually occurs between the ages of 45 and 55. In some cases periods become scanty and infrequent at this time, without undue discomfort, before ceasing altogether; whilst in others there is considerable menstrual upset. An interval of six months amenorrhoea is considered definitive and bleeding after this needs urgent referral to a gynaecologist for investigation of post-menopausal bleeding (PMB). For full security, whichever method of contraception is in force should be continued for a further year after the menopause. If there is any doubt FSH levels in blood can be checked to confirm a lack of ability to ovulate.

Knowledge of the changes occurring at the menopause will assist the nurse in understanding the woman's problems and may enable her to anticipate some of the questions. Because the population is living longer most women will survive the menopause by a considerable number of years and because of substantial alteration in the attitudes shown towards the need for adequate therapy there is no reason why any woman should suffer unnecessarily from menopausal symptoms.

Some women approach the menopause with misgivings as they see the end of their reproductive capabilities approaching. Others are heartened by the impending release from the turmoil of menstruation and the fear of unexpected pregnancy. A great deal has been written about the menopause and discussed on television and radio, and most of this has encouraged enquiry about the benefits of hormone replacement therapy (HRT). In fact few women suffer severe symptoms and many notice no appreciable change in their lifestyle. However, those who are unlucky enough to suffer serious symptoms should receive sympathetic support and adequate treatment after full investigation.

Menopausal symptoms

The symptoms which cause the most distress are related to the withdrawal of oestrogen. The main symptoms are hot flushes and attacks of sweating, especially at night. The frequency of the attacks may be easily tolerated, but if they occur so often as to cause social embarrassment then they may make life an absolute misery, with broken concentration and worry when a busy job is constantly interrupted.

Another common difficulty is associated with a dry vagina which makes intercourse uncomfortable. Without the effect of oestrogen the skin of the vagina becomes thin and sensitive and the normal vaginal secretions and moisture in the vagina are very much reduced. Döderlein's bacilli are unable to thrive in their normal numbers and the acidity of the vagina is therefore reduced, leaving it much more susceptible to infection. The atrophic changes can be treated with local applications of oestrogen cream which usually alleviates the problem. Women with this symptom should be carefully and gently examined to be sure that the vagina is not excoriated or infected.

Some women will complain of reduced libido. This needs careful discussion as it may be due to discomfort or to psycho-sexual anxieties such as the fear of being less attractive; or there may be marital disharmony. Poor concentration and memory sometimes associated with fatigue is a frequent complaint. These may not be entirely menopausal in origin, but the result of tension and anxiety and with treatment they may improve as other symptoms improve. Osteoporosis, honeycombing of the bony skeleton, is common in postmenopausal women, when the loss of circulating oestrogen causes the bones to become fragile and more liable to fracture. Although some women will only suffer minor changes, many will benefit from HRT which if commenced before bone changes have occurred will halt the decalcification process.

Menopause medication

Hot flushes may respond to various non-hormonal preparations. The overactivity of the skin capillaries in response to massive amounts of circulating FSH can be influenced by small doses of phenobarbitone or clonidine, 0.05 mg twice daily. There is also considerable enthusiasm for preparations containing oil of evening primrose, and Royal Jelly has its supporters.

Whilst combined oral contraceptives would supply more than adequate hormone replacement therapy it is usual to prescribe special preparations. Premarin is a conjugated oestrogen which is obtained from horses and more exactly mimics the natural human substance, but it is possible to use synthetic oestrogen such as ethinyl oestradiol either in tablet form or as a subcutaneous implant. There is another synthetic oral preparation which contains oestradiol valerate. It is quite important that oestrogens are not given by themselves except after hysterectomy as the unopposed oestrogen may have a carcinogenic effect on the endometrium lining the womb. For this reason it is usual to give some progestogen for part of each month, and this should provoke a withdrawal bleed similar to a period. When it is safe to give oestrogen alone it is possible to use the recently developed skin-patch system which consists of a small sticky plaster with a special coating to allow measured amounts of hormone to be absorbed through the adjacent skin. It needs to be applied twice weekly and is very convenient to use. Oestrogen replacement therapy ought to result in regular withdrawal bleeding (except after hysterectomy) and should this be disrupted then the woman must be aware that she needs to seek further advice without delay.

14.4 THE HANDICAPPED AND DISABLED

The aim of this section is to make health professionals aware of the needs of handicapped people in achieving a satisfactory sexual relationship. Nurses are very often the first to be approached by a patient about sexual problems, and their attitudes and informed support will encourage a physically disabled person to make the adaptations to their restrictions. People regard sexual relationships as an intimate and very personal part of their lives and if there are physical disabilities it will take courage to discuss them. Health professionals working in all areas constantly come across people who have become disabled as a result of accidents, surgery or illness. In these circumstances if supportive efforts are made to encourage open discussion with the individual then a more confident attitude towards his or her sexual and reproductive capability will develop.

It is more common to find that contraceptive advice is offered to disabled people either by the domiciliary family planning team or the general practitioner. The practical difficulties of getting to a clinic and the anxiety of meeting other people attending for contraceptive advice whose initial attitude may show incredulity is too daunting and inclined to reduce their motivation. Health professionals should be aware that individual advice for disabled people may be obtained by contacting specialist organizations such as the Multiple Sclerosis Society and others.

Causes of disability vary widely and fall naturally into three broad groups according to the degree of incapacity.

Conditions which may impair sexual relationships although there is potentially normal sexual function

● Disfigurement which causes embarrassment such as severe scarring from burns, birthmarks, mastectomy, general surgery and amputation.
● Limitation of physical exertion due to angina, heart disease, asthma, bronchitis, other lung disease and hernia.
● Early limitation of movement in progressive disease such as muscular dystrophy and multiple sclerosis.
● Discomfort during intercourse due to early arthritis, abdominal and vaginal surgery, and unstable spinal pain.

Conditions causing reduced sexual function

Impairment may be due to a lack of muscle power or co-ordination, and such conditions include spasticity, paraplegia, quadraplegia, severe spinal damage or spina bifida. Men may be unable to achieve an adequate erection where the sympathetic and para-sympathetic nerve supply is interfered with by hypertensive drug therapy or surgical interruption; for instance during aortic grafting procedures. Prostatectomy by abdominal operation frequently disrupts the ejaculatory duct and although erection is not impaired intercourse will rarely climax with ejaculation and procreation is therefore unlikely.

Conditions which impair communication

This category includes the blind or partially sighted, the deaf or partially deaf, those with severe speech defects, mental retardation, and some forms of mental illness.

It would be rash to assume that any of these conditions are invariably areas of concern. The nurse should always enquire indirectly about the restrictions and problems envisaged by the particular person before attempting to make any helpful sugges-tions. Many people with handicaps are so well adjusted to their restrictions that they do not consider they have problems and will be disconcerted to learn that other people view them differently. Alternatively, others with relatively minor restrictions may be less adaptable and find themselves unable to cope with their new image, and they will need a great deal of counselling and support to make adaptations. The degree of difficulty is that which the individual sees for him or herself. Conditions arising from birth will often be seen quite differently from those acquired suddenly. Congenital disabilities give rise to the additional consideration such as the advisability of having children who may inherit the condition. These anxieties should be explored with the couple concerned and referrals for genetic counselling should be arranged when this becomes appropriate. Some women whose lives may be severely at risk should pregnancy occur need to be clearly told about the urgent need for effective contraception from a well informed source.

Friends, relatives and partners are all involved in the long term happiness of the handicapped person and in some cases it may help to include them in a frank discussion about the need and availability of help and advice on sexual matters. This is an area which calls for the services of people specially trained to work with special problems of the disabled and there are courses available for those who wish to develop these skills. Individual societies for particular illnesses have services for offering advice and these can be contacted through the Committee on Sexual and Personal Relationships of the Disabled (SPOD, 286 Camden Road, London N7). This organization has a network of counsellors and produces literature to cover most physical disabilities.

14.5 DRUG ABUSE AND CONTRACEPTION

Low priority is given to the use of contraception by many drug addicts and those who do request advice are likely to be erratic in motivation. In many cases the woman receives contraceptive advice for the first time in a post termination environment.

Careful consideration of the client's lifestyle is necessary if any satisfactory outcome is to be obtained. Many drug addicts have irregular periods or amenorrhoea and may be infertile since heroin can suppress ovulation. Ovulation, however, does return within a few months of withdrawal of heroin, and with other drugs may occur spasmodically. In addition dietary deficiencies may result in anorexic type problems with ovulation.

Oral contraception may be satisfactory for some drug abusers who still lead a reasonably controlled existence, but in many cases the erratic lifestyle coupled with the high incidence of liver damage and hepatitis make oral contraception a poor choice.

Intrauterine devices need to be carefully considered especially if there is any possibility of prostitution being used as a means of subsidizing the high cost of addiction. Barrier methods, especially sheaths and spermicides, are the safest and most favoured methods, but as they require motivation it is highly likely that they will not be used consistently. Recently, the publicity regarding AIDS has however boosted the use of this latter method and any effective method is to be encouraged in view of the effects that drugs of addiction have on a developing pregnancy.

14.6 PEOPLE FROM OTHER COUNTRIES

The population of Britain is now so multinational that it becomes necessary for health professionals to have some insight into the particular views held by people from other cultures if they are to understand their different customs and provide them with effective advice on contraception when it is sought. Unfortunately, because of the immense scope of the subject, it is possible only to deal rather superficially with the special needs of some minority groups who now live permanently in this country, and we are all too conscious that the details given are regrettably more generalized than we would like. It is hoped, however, that they provide an introduction which may stimulate clinic personnel to look in greater depth at the interesting cultural traditions and customs of the immigrant population they are most likely to meet in clinics and to acquire some understanding of certain basic beliefs which influence attitudes to contraception.

Immigrant families newly arrived in this country are faced with many radical changes in their accustomed way of life and tend to cling for a while to their old-established customs. Health staff who have worked in their countries of origin will, from their own experience, appreciate only too well the extent of the upheaval involved. As the families adapt to the English way of life their views will gradually change. This could mean that some ambivalent feelings might emerge about the use of contraception, especially if this subject was not open for discussion at home. The nurse must establish with individuals what their views are and endeavour to provide them with clear information about the methods available so that they can choose with confidence a method that they will find acceptable.

Communication may be difficult if there is a language barrier. Special literature in a number of languages is provided from various sources and this should be freely available at clinics. It is possible to get the services of many excellent interpreters, and some people bring an English-speaking friend or relative to the clinic to help them. However, it is always tricky to work through a third party whose attitude may unintentionally distort the information relayed, and sometimes information may be misinterpreted. In a few clinics, staff and interpreters have combined forces to produce tape recordings of general information on contraception which can be used individually by non English-speaking people while waiting in the clinic. This releases the interpreter to work in more depth with the individual woman when she is being seen by the nurse or doctor after she has had time to absorb the information given on the tape recorder. It is hoped that this system might be extended to overcome language problems in all appropriate family planning clinics. The influence of friends and family is often far more important to the immigrant couple than the information received from a doctor. The nurse must attempt to establish a good enough rapport to make sure that where external pressures exist, she will be able to listen with understanding and help the woman to come to terms with the changes which confront her whole way of life.

A wide variety of Asian people from several parts of the Indian sub-continent and East Africa now live in this country and form a large proportion of those attending clinics. There is a wide range of attitudes and responses from them regarding family planning. Some Asian girls who have been born and educated in this country will be prepared to use contraception while developing a marital relationship, or to space their children after marriage. Some families retain their traditional customs and would never consider contraception, believing it to be an unacceptable interference with the pattern of life. Between these two extremes there are many families who find that the social and economic differences in western life force them to reconsider their traditional customs. Many Asians, especially those from rural areas, have a very different pattern of family life. They live in an extended family environment often very close physically to each other. The extended family has a strict code of behaviour for the mutual benefit and safety of all its members. The hierarchical structure within the family increases with age, and though often equal, the roles of men and women are clearly defined. The daughters marry into their husband's family and thereafter are supported, cared for and advised by the women in his family circle. The subject of sex, and child-rearing, is the business of married women, and they help and advise each other within the family. There is little sex education of any kind outside this unit, nor is it provided during attendance at school, so general knowledge on this subject is slight. Asian women are modest and rarely discuss matters of contraception or sexual problems. The subject is so private that husband and wife may not have discussed the matter themselves, and it would be unthinkable to do so with a strange third party. Community health staff and family planning teams who provide contraceptive advice for some of these families have to approach the subject delicately.

Contraception is not necessarily required by all couples. They may wish to follow traditional customs and have several children. However, in their own country the proximity of the extended family provides assistance with other children and household duties while the new arrival settles into the family: here, they may be coping alone. In their homeland breast feeding is more common, and this will contribute to wider spacing of children, some of whom, sadly, will not survive. In this country many women bottle feed their babies and there is a lower infant mortality rate which will contribute to a larger, more closely spaced family. If the woman is also assisting her husband as bread-winner, the social and economic pressures will force them to reconsider their views about not limiting family size. The extended family, which continues to be influential and supportive even when fragmented by emigration, may be asked for advice concerning restriction of family size. These decisions will then be made, often very imaginatively and with understanding by a more senior woman in the family, but even if the advice conflicts with the satellite family's needs, it will not usually be overridden. This fact will be useful for a nurse who is involved in helping with contraceptive advice as there may be considerable guilt and ambivalence about using contraception if there is conflict about its acceptability. It will take some women longer than others to make decisions of this sort for themselves.

A wide variety of religions are practised among the minority groups living in this country, many of which are so interrelated with daily customs of living that it becomes difficult to know which customs are based in religion and which in cultural traditions. In either case they command obedience about particular social behaviour which is keenly adhered to and sensitive to disruption. If the nurse is aware of some of the implications that contraception and its possible side effects may have for a family, she may find it easier to help them more effectively to find an acceptable method of contraception.

It is always worth while enquiring whether the person requesting contraception is prepared to be seen and examined by a male doctor. In some cases there may be strong preferences for male doctors. However, a few women are less embarrassed by another woman, and some cultures forbid a woman to be touched by any man other than her husband. If this is the case it would be best, except in cases of emergency, to direct the couple to a clinic in which a female doctor is usually available.

Another area which may cause concern is that of menstrual disturbance. Menstrual loss is considered by some to be unclean. Certain cultures will not permit women to prepare food when they are menstruating, nor have intercourse until after a ritual bath. Intercourse may not be practised during menstruation. If the chosen method of contraception produces menstrual irregularity it is unlikely to be acceptable, and may cause considerable offence to the social arrangements.

The use of injections of hormonal preparations is emotive in some groups of immigrants while others are delighted with it. Should it become more widely used, great care should be taken that it is never used for a woman without very clear informed consent which should be recorded in the case notes when obtained.

Some women are very modest and may find the practical problems of getting sufficient privacy to insert a cap a deterrent in its effective use. Some cultures allow a woman to use only her left hand when touching her genital area, the right hand being preserved as 'clean'. In this case the nurse must teach the woman to insert a cap with the left hand only, if the method is to be successfully adopted. This will entail adapting the teaching of cap insertion to exclude the use of spermicide on both surfaces which will make it less slippery to handle. The cervical surface should have the spermicide, as usual, and additional spermicide in the form of a pessary can be inserted after the cap is in place.

Male barrier methods could often be acceptable in a male dominated household. Even Rastafarians, a group who seldom use contraception, may find it acceptable to use condoms providing they are black.

In some cultures it is important that the woman is a virgin at her marriage. It is important that if these women should seek pre-marital contraceptive advice the routine vaginal examination is not carried out even if it is found to be necessary.

Unplanned pregnancy is usually associated with stressful decisions, but some cultures impose on women a strong urge to prove their fertility. This has led to a more relaxed attitude amongst these women about having children out of wedlock. The nurse should be aware that a woman may be delighted for this reason to have conceived but may not necessarily wish to continue with the pregnancy. There may also be considerable resistance, even after more than one pregnancy, to consider contraception. On other occasions the traditions of the family may be stretched to breaking point if a girl becomes pregnant out of wedlock, as it brings shame to all the family members. Expulsion from the family may be one of the dire consequences, and this will leave the girl totally unsupported and desperate. This is the type of problem which requires the utmost help and long term support by a social worker.

Roman Catholic couples can receive advice from the Catholic Advisory Bureau about spacing their pregnancies by natural methods. This type of advice is similar to that which can be offered at clinics, but is related to avoiding, rather than preventing, a pregnancy.

Women from North America, Australia and Scandinavia who are resident in this country also attend clinics in quite large numbers. Their requests for advice and examination are less often complicated by language problems, but their direct approach and lack of inhibitions can sometimes surprise the nurse by their outspoken comments.

15

Fertility problems

There are a variety of opinions about when help should be sought by a couple apparently unable to conceive. Various figures are quoted on normal rates of conception, and these range from 65% to 90% in the first year following the discontinuance of contraceptive measures. It is reasonable to suppose that the average couple should have achieved pregnancy within 18 months. It is difficult for a young couple to understand that having taken precautions to prevent a pregnancy there may then be a delay before they can actually start a family. If they have been receiving contraceptive advice it seems unlikely that there will be problems with non-consummation, but enquiries should be made about sexual difficulties.

Most people attending the clinic are thoroughly aware of the time in their cycle when they are most likely to ovulate so they are unlikely to be missing the fertile phase. An enquiry about this, however, is not inappropriate and by virtue of their training, family planning nurses will be aware of the fertile phase which is 14 days before the onset of the next menstrual period. Fertility decreases with age in women and if she has taken contraceptive precautions for a number of years it is possible that because she is older, she will need to be exposed to more episodes of intercourse at just the right time to achieve a pregnancy. This is not the case with men whose sperm retain the facility to fertilize whatever their age.

15.1 SELF-HELP FOR DELAY IN CONCEIVING

The fertile phase has already been mentioned, but there are other things which the couple can do to increase the chances of conceiving. Semen has to be in close contact with the cervix, for the sperm must be able to to get through the external os and into the cervical canal. Where a uterus is known to be retroverted it may be difficult for the semen to make contact with the external os and so it is a good idea if, following intercourse, the woman props her buttocks up on a pillow or over her partner's legs.

Spermatozoa are best formed at a temperature fractionally below that which is usual for the body; this is why the testicles are found outside the abdomen. The wearing of tight clothing and underwear in particular may increase the temperature so that the sperm count is not as high as it could be. It may therefore be advisable for the male partner to give up wearing support underwear for something a little looser, but this will have to be the norm for two or three months before any effect is noticed as the sperm take this long to go through the process of formation.

15.2 FIRST ENQUIRIES INTO THE INABILITY TO CONCEIVE

The best time to commence investigations into the failure of a couple to conceive usually turns out to be after about 12 months of unprotected intercourse. If the woman is over 30 years of age, 6 months may be realistic and where the woman is approaching the menopause it may be necessary to act immediately so that no valuable time is lost. Investigation of the couple must rest with fertility experts and this usually means that the initial approach is made by the family doctor to an interested gynaecologist. Once a firm diagnosis has been made other specialists may become involved. Specialist investigations cover four main questions:

1. Is the woman ovulating and ovulating well;
2. Are her fallopian tubes patent;
3. Is the man producing satisfactory quantities of normal motile sperm;
4. Are the sperm to be found in the right place at the right time so that they are able to fertilize the ovum?

The first visit to a gynaecologist entails an interview and medical examination, preferably of both partners. Decisions are then made about the necessity for tests. Many questions will occur to the couple and it is helpful if a properly informed nurse can be available to clarify the advice given and be able to deal with any questions arising from the interview. A fertility history is very personal, and time and sensitivity are essential factors if vital information is not to be missed. The nurse can contribute to a successful interview by ensuring that there is no interruption and that the appointments allow sufficient time to muster all the facts and provide explanation.

15.3 THE HISTORY

The aim of the first interview is to obtain a full history, to provide a picture of the couple's sexual and emotional relationships, their ages, time since marriage and how long they have been having unprotected intercourse. It occasionally becomes evident that intercourse has never taken place properly or may be such an infrequent event that there has not been a reasonable chance for a pregnancy to occur. If this is the case the couple may only require supportive advice to achieve a successful outcome. Psycho-sexual difficulties may come to light for one or other partner or even both of them and these will require proper counselling and quite often need referal to a psychotherapist.

Details of the family history and social and religious background are important. There may be parental pressure on a couple to reproduce. This type of psychological pressure from family or friends can cause considerable tension which contributes to a lack of success. Occasionally the underlying factor for the distress is the shame and embarrassment of appearing barren or impotent and if the couple are both found to be capable of fertilization they may live quite happily secure in the fact that their childlessness is not related to a personal abnormality.

The occupations of both partners should be recorded as it sometimes transpires that there are hurdles such as shift work or frequent physical separation to account for the difficulties. Sperm production is very sensitive to temperature and as has already been discussed the position of the testicles in the scrotum is designed to keep their environment cool. If the man spends a great deal of time sitting, for example as a professional driver, the temperature will be higher than optimum with resulting restriction in the manufacture of sperm. A similar effect occurs with chefs and other men who have to endure a hot working environment. This problem can be intensified if the man wears close fitting under-pants or tight jeans which by themselves can interfere quite enough with sperm manufacture to radically reduce the output.

For successful fertilization a large number of sperm are necessary to support the one lucky sperm in achieving its objective, so reduced numbers are a significant stumbling block.

The man's medical history may reveal an undescended testis which may have suffered damage if it was not surgically rescued from the inguinal canal before puberty. Other surgery involving the repair of a hernia could have damaged the vas where it passes through the inguinal canal. Epididymo-orchitis (testicular inflammation) can result in permanent damage to the sperm-making machinery, especially when it is caused by mumps. Other infections of the epididymis can also have a similar effect. Smoking and alcohol in excess can reduce the fertility without necessarily being at all obvious so they should always be enquired about.

The female history commences with details of the menstrual cycle, its regularity and frequency being of particular interest. It is important to discover if the woman understands the probable time of ovulation in relation to her period and how she should use this to time intercourse. Inquiries are also made about any relevant medical conditions; for instance, thyroid imbalance or pelvic inflammatory disease. A particularly messy appendicitis with a ruptured appendix can be the start of a pelvic infection which results in tubal blockage. Smoking seems to have an effect in the same way as it does with the male partner and should be actively discouraged. This will have the additional benefit that if a pregnancy is achieved the fetus will not have to suffer the assaults of nicotine.

15.4 EXAMINATION

Both partners should be encouraged to come on the first visit so that dual responsibility is taken right from the outset and a comprehensive start may speed progress.

The male external genitalia are observed and abnormalities of the penis such as hypospadias eliminated. Where the man is uncircumcized the prepuce should be drawn back to ascertain whether there is any phimosis (tightening of the foreskin) and inflammation or discharge. The size and consistency of both testicles is assessed by palpation and any tenderness noted, especially of the epididymis. Finally both groins should be examined for the presence of herniorraphy scars or actual herniae. If a testicle is absent from the scrotal sac it should be sought in the inguinal canal.

Female examination follows the pattern already described in Chapter 6 with special attention being paid to secondary sexual development.

15.5 INVESTIGATIONS INTO FERTILITY

Male investigations

Semen analysis
This provides information about the total numbers of sperm; their appearance and how many abnormal forms appear; as well as their mobility. Local laboratory services will have their own particular requirements and a test should not be arranged without first ascertaining what these are as well as the times for delivery of the sample.

It is usually recommended that the man abstains from ejaculation for three days before the semen is collected by masturbation. When this is impossible coitus interruptus can be attempted but it is quite likely that the first fraction of the ejaculate could be lost and as it is particularly rich in sperm the count may be misleadingly low. Collection in a condom is unsatisfactory because of the chemicals used in finishing the rubber product. Additionally some brands are coated with a spermicide.

Agglutination may be observed and should be suspected if the count appears to be unusually high. The average fertile specimen with a volume of 2–5 ml has a sperm density of between 40 and 100 million sperm per cubic centimetre. It is usual for the laboratory to look for sperm antibodies, especially when agglutination has been noted. The presence of pus cells is suggestive of infection and cultures will be set up when necessary to search for the causative organism.

Where large numbers of abnormal sperm are identified it may be necessary to check the male chromosome karyotype. A low sperm count (oligospermia) or complete absence of sperm (azoospermia) require examination to find out if there is testicular abnormality or related varicocele. Other tests involving the male partner are made to exclude imbalance of hormone levels which would affect spermatogenesis. Levels of follicle stimulating hormone, luteinizing hormone and testosterone are estimated from blood samples. Occasionally further samples to measure prolactin levels and adrenocortical hormone levels are also made.

Joint investigations

Post-coital test

This is a very useful method of determining that the sperm are being delivered to the right place and are able to gain entry into the receptive cervical canal. Intercourse should take place between four and twelve hours prior to the woman's appointment and she should be instructed not to take a bath or douche herself before she is examined. It is essential that this test is only carried out when ovulation is expected so that the sample of mucus aspirated from the cervical canal is not too sticky for the sperm to swim through it. The aspirated mucus is examined under a microscope and the number of progressively motile sperm is identified.

Crossed hostility test

This test is performed when there is reason to believe that a substance hostile to sperm is present in the cervical mucus. The test, similar to the post-coital test, involves examining the motility and behaviour of the partner's sperm and donor sperm in an aspirated specimen of ovulatory cervical mucus. The woman should abstain from intercourse for three days before the test and should be accompanied by her partner so that a fresh semen sample is available. Both tests are carried out under the microscope and involve separately comparing the penetration and motility of donor and partner's sperm in the divided sample of cervical mucus.

Female investigations

In the absence of any obvious anatomical abnormalities of the external genitalia, investigations should centre on whether ovulation is occurring in the normal way. The simplest method is to estimate the basal body temperature, and it is recommended that a digital thermometer is obtained. The temperature is recorded on waking and before moving about so that it more closely represents the basal sleeping levels. A rise should occur at or about ovulation but minor pyrexia can cause difficulty in identifying this alteration. Each day the measurements are entered on a chart which includes the menstrual calendar and times when intercourse took place. It cannot be too strongly stated that the test must be properly explained so that the information is as reliable as possible, and in order to avoid unnecessary anxiety it is best to make it short and accurate, lasting for three to six cycles.

Serum progesterone levels can be expected to be significantly raised 7 days after ovulation and a blood sample is usually obtained on day 21 (where the cycle is 28 days) to confirm that ovulation has taken place. In longer cycles the test needs to be appropriately delayed. The progestogenic effect can be identified in the cellular appearance of the endometrium and occasionally an endometrial biopsy is undertaken, usually at the same time as tubal patency tests. The LH surge which appears in the blood just prior to ovulation is the basis for the various ovulation prediction kits which have recently become available from retail pharmacists. Early morning urine specimens can be tested daily or every other day around the time of ovulation for LH levels and a simple colour change indicates the event. Many women have already made their own preliminary investigation by this method.

In the absence of regular menstruation it may be necessary to estimate FSH as well as LH in the woman's blood. Prolactin may be raised because of a pituitary adenoma or more usually for no very clear reason. The first elevated level should be checked in case it has been artificially raised by stress, but if this is not the case then a pituitary fossa X-ray is necessary to exclude tumour. Blood tests are also undertaken to assess normal thyroid function. Blood oestrogen levels are necessary to identify the correct method of stimulating ovulation.

The investigation of tubal patency is most satisfactorily achieved by laparoscopy. The insertion of an optical system through the umbilicus under a general anaesthetic allows the pelvic organs to be visualized, and the passage of dye injected through the cervix confirms patency of the system when it spills out from the fimbrial ends of the tubes. Where the corpus luteum is identified on one of the ovaries ovulation can be assumed and inactive or polycystic ovaries can be biopsied. A general view of the pelvis does sometimes reveal endometriosis which if severe may obstruct fertilization. Occasionally, even if this may be so mild as to preclude mechanical disadvantage it can still delay successful conception. Use of intrauterine injection of radio-opaque dye in conjunction with X-ray image intensification is known as hysterosalpingography. This occupies a less important place now that laparoscopy is easily available. It does have a place in identifying intrauterine septa and congenital abnormalities of the reproductive

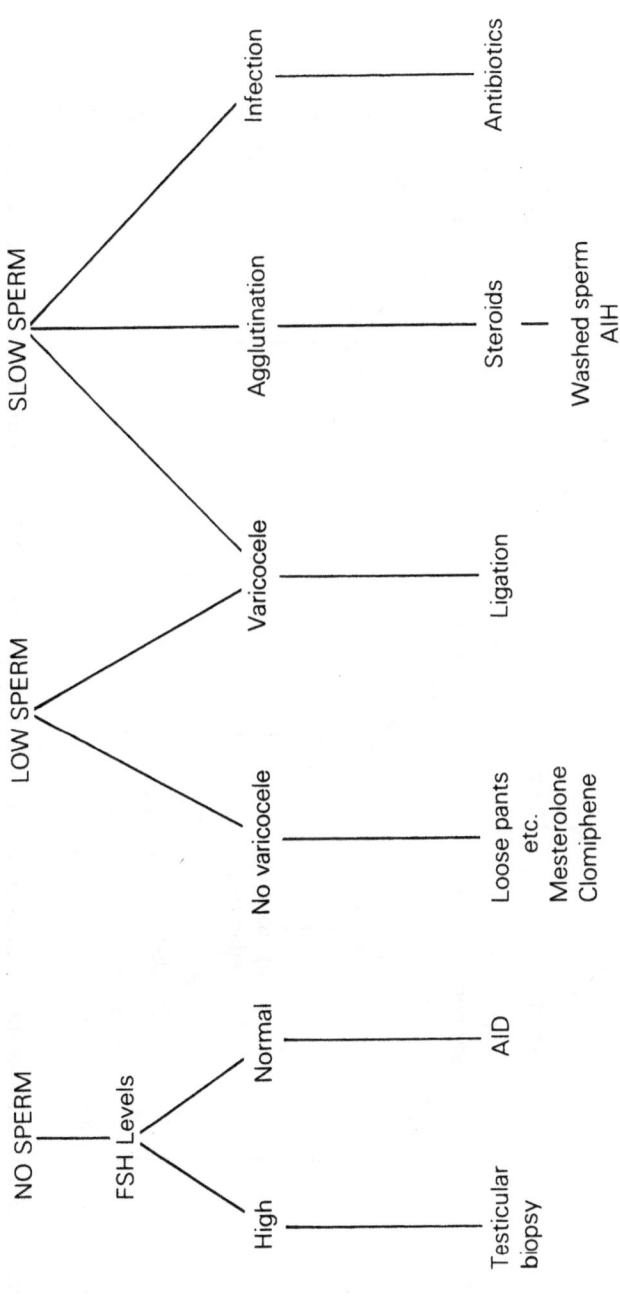

Figure 15.1 Chart showing treatment of basic male fertility problems. AID = artificial insemination by donor; AIH = artificial insemination by husband.

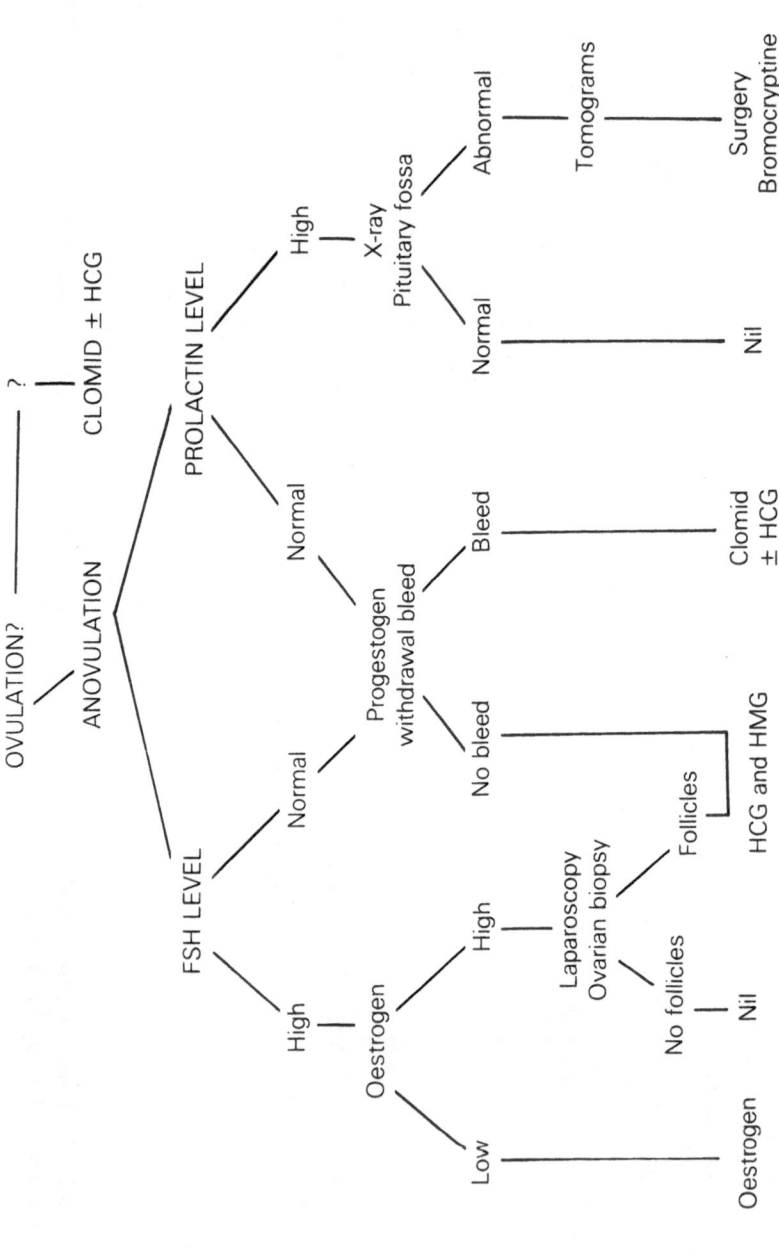

Figure 15.2 Chart showing treatment of female fertility problems. HCG = human chorionic gonadotrophin; HMG = human menopause gonadotrophin. HMG may be raised if weight loss is extreme and ovulation impaired.

organs. Whilst it has usually been carried out as an out-patient procedure the discomfort that it produces should not be under-estimated. Women should be accompanied if possible for this twenty minute procedure by their partner or a friend.

15.6 TREATMENT

Male and female treatments are diagrammatically expressed in Figures 15.1 and 15.2 respectively.

15.7 PSYCHOLOGICAL ASPECTS

Considerable psychological pressure is placed on a couple under-going investigation for subfertility, so some thought and prep-aration prior to seeking consultant advice is worthwhile. There is about equal chance that either may be the infertile member of the relationship although there is also a possibility that no obvious reason is identified after exhaustive investigation. The psycho-logical and social implication of the results on both individuals of infertility might benefit from some meditation in advance. They will then be in a better position to cope with their own reactions and those of their family. They need to aim at developing firm loving support and understanding if the best results are to be obtained.

16

Pre-pregnancy care

Family planning nurses are in an ideal position to help women to avoid unnecessary risks during childbearing. It is common sense if a pregnancy is planned that both parents should be in the best of health and avoid substances that are likely to damage the fetus such as alcohol, certain drugs, smoking and a polluted environment. A few couples have existing risks which cannot be removed although they may be modified by having expert opinion and supervision before embarking on a pregnancy. When clients first attend the family planning clinic a full history is obtained, and from this various risks for future healthy childbearing may emerge. It is helpful in these cases to inform the woman even at this stage that when she contemplates having a family it would be wise to see her doctor or an appropriate specialist six months or more beforehand for advice and assessment.

The woman is not alone in needing pre-pregnancy discussion: the partner also needs to consider his health and social behaviour. Smoking, excess alcohol and drug abuse in either partner present a hazard to a potential pregnancy. Abnormal sperm formation has been shown to be associated with lead pollution at work.

16.1 DIETARY FACTORS

The pregnant mother's body undergoes rapid changes once fertilization has taken place, and the physiological needs of a developing baby are met well in advance of its demands. A vital safety factor rests with having really good nourishment for as long as possible beforehand because if the dietary history is good the effect of teratogenic agents, where they exist, is greatly reduced. Dieting, nutritional restrictions of cultural origin and severe dietary abuse should be noted by the nurse, as well as any illness which may have contributed to poor nourishment. In severe cases such as anorexia nervosa ovulation is impaired, returning as the condition improves. Research shows that it is hazardous to start a pregnancy before the body has a chance of replenishing its stores and this may take a year or more. Dietary abuse results not only in the depletion of those foodstuffs concerned with energy and tissue growth but also of trace elements which are essential if the fetus is to develop in the normal way and avoid spontaneous abortion or perinatal death. Nurses should take the time to discuss the woman's normal eating habits, her economic constraints, cultural restraints and personal lifestyle so that advice can be given about anything from a minor adjustment to seeking specialist advice.

16.2 GENERAL HEALTH

A family history of congenital abnormality or unexplained stillbirth may lead to anxiety about inherited disorders, and whilst this may be within the scope of some general practitioners it could be that referral to a specialist in genetic counselling would be appropriate.

Any of the more severe long term medical conditions may come to light during the initial interview, such as cardiac disease, diabetes or thyroid imbalance. These can give rise to additional anxiety during reproduction and because of the rapid increase in circulating fluid which occurs in pregnancy, any past illness or present disease involving heart, lungs, kidneys or liver will need medical assessment. In cardiac disease the main risk is directly related to the increase in maternal blood volume and the ability of the heart to increase its output by 50% in the first half of pregnancy. Practical problems related to physical strain will include the ability to continue work, care for young children, cope with domestic duties and negotiate stairs.

In some circumstances a medical condition may cause not only maternal ill-health but also affect the fetal development. In diabetic mothers it has been shown that the risks of subfertility, miscarriage, stillbirth and congenital abnormality are raised when the condition is not well controlled at the time of conception.

Sometimes the woman may have one of the conditions which require regular medication, for example epilepsy or psychiatric illness, and whilst this may not adversely affect the baby the drugs may not be acceptable. These may need to be stopped or changed before embarking on pregnancy. Treatment for thyrotoxicosis with antithyroid drugs should continue when the mother is pregnant; however there is a theoretical risk of suppressing the fetal thyroid and this is avoided by giving the mother a small dose of thyroxine. Due to increasing metabolism throughout pregnancy most medication will need to be reviewed at regular intervals.

The woman who appears to be pale and clinically anaemic, or whose history suggests chronic blood loss, may benefit from an haemoglobin estimation. Where indicated, iron therapy perhaps with additional vitamins can then be prescribed before embarking on a pregnancy when they are more reliably absorbed. Extra supplements of some vitamins may have the undesired effects of reducing the natural ability of the body to absorb other elements, such as zinc, which could prove more important for the safety of the pregnancy. Natural body adjustment will occur if the diet is satisfactory and this must be the safest way to rectify any depletion in the stores.

16.3 OBSTETRIC HISTORY

Women who have experienced a successful outcome to a previous pregnancy always recall their relief that all went well. Very few enter a subsequent pregnancy without some anxiety about the safety of the venture. A few less fortunate women will have had bad experiences and require reassurance and advice aimed at mitigating or avoiding a similar problem. Some obstetric problems can be modified and even prevented with a little anticipation and therefore timely and accurate advice is important.

Any loss of a previous pregnancy will give distress whether it was caused by the decision to terminate the pregnancy or if it was spontaneously aborted. Anxiety is stimulated concerning the future loss of a pregnancy and fears are often very deep and difficult to express, particularly if there is a perceived fault to overcome. Couples who have had a single spontaneous abortion can be reassured that there is optimistic statistical evidence to support the successful outcome of a subsequent pregnancy. Even a second miscarriage hardly weighs the odds unfavourably but recurrent abortion warrants further investigation before attempting a further pregnancy. Semen analysis may show increased numbers of abnormal forms of sperm and karyotyping the blood of both parents can reveal chromosome abnormalities in up to 50% of investigations.

If a known genetically transmitted condition exists in the family history then the partners should be encouraged to consult their family practitioner who will in most cases refer the matter to a specialist genetic centre where advice about an ever-extending range of conditions can be obtained. Much of this advice will be based on information about incidents which have occurred amongst relatives. Some of these conditions are only important if they are carried by both parents. An example of this is sickle cell disease where only minimal effects are present in the carrier or trait state. In other circumstances only one parent may be responsible for an hereditary abnormality.

Pregnancy occurring in the older age group has a higher incidence of morbidity and mortality for both mother and infant, so although it is less likely to occur, a pregnancy near the menopause must be managed very carefully. Early ante-natal booking and screening with consultant supervision is necessary. Maternal age at the extremes of female reproductive ability gives cause for concern. Spontaneously occurring chromosomal abnormalities (i.e. without any family history) are seen more often among the under-twenties, whilst over the age of 35 the frequency increases with each succeeding year.

Abnormalities in the structure of the reproductive organs, such as fibroids which are large enough to distort the uterine cavity, or a bicornute uterus interfering with normal function, may provoke miscarriages until the anatomy is surgically modified. Later loss of pregnancy in the absence of any abnormality of the uterine cavity may be due to incompetence of the internal os or of the cervix. This circular muscle needs to support the pressure of the developing pregnancy and where there is a history of spontaneous abortion after 14 weeks' gestation or very premature delivery a purse-string suture can be inserted in the cervix to provide extra strength. Early miscarriage following termination is unlikely to be caused by the previous operation but if the event occurs after 12 weeks' gestation gynaecological advice should be sought.

Bacterial, viral and protozoal infections can damage or abort a pregnancy. The effects of the rubella virus are well documented and family planning clinics should be on the lookout for non-immune individuals well before they embark on pregnancy. Blood testing for rubella antibodies will pick up those women at risk who can then be offered vaccination. 'Flu epidemics and other viral infections may be associated with early loss of pregnancy. Whilst this may also happen with a primary attack of genital herpes,

chronic infections may infect the neonate during vaginal delivery
by contamination from the birth canal. The interval of inactivity
between attacks of herpes tends to lengthen which will allow safe
vaginal delivery in those cases where negative cultures from
cervical swabs and an absence of any genital lesions exist at the end
of pregnancy. Bacterial infection is especially common in the
female urinary tract and may be asymptomatic. Acute urinary
infections may develop and as these are able to ascend from the
bladder to the kidneys and cause severe pyelitis any history of
infection needs to be treated without delay. In middle to late
pregnancy this is a common cause of premature uterine activity
which may result in fetal loss or an immature baby.

Premature delivery of the baby, whatever the cause, has a
tendency to recur and every opportunity should be taken to
attempt to avoid it happening by providing close supervision in
successive pregnancies, since premature infants do not always
develop as satisfactorily as their mature counterparts.

Operative intervention

A number of women who have had previous confinements
requiring operative intervention come for pre-conceptual counselling to allay their fears about history repeating itself. Whilst
explanations were almost certainly given at the time, the ability to
absorb and retain information is always impaired at a time of crisis,
and quite frequently needs repeating and reinforcing. Further
clarification ought to increase their confidence especially where
records indicate a non-recurring episode. Sometimes vigorous
requests for particular methods of management have conflicted
with the outcome and the couple became bewildered and angry. It
is of the utmost importance that the confidence of the couple to
cope with future pregnancies in an effective and positive way is
kept in mind throughout the interview. Those women who have
recently experienced a caesarean section need to be informed that
they should not contemplate a further pregnancy until the scar
tissue in the uterus is firmly healed. This requires individual advice
and is usually a minimum of nine months.

16.4 IMMUNIZATION

There is no evidence that immunization against influenza, cholera and poliomyelitis causes damage to the fetus. It is a good general rule, however, to restrict administration to women who have strong indications for protection and it is prudent even then to avoid the first trimester. Wherever possible it would seem sensible to avoid conception for three months after any immunization.

Rubella

Although this is a mild disease its consequence on the sight, hearing, brain and heart development of the fetus may be devastating if the mother contracts the infection, particularly in early pregnancy. It would seem good practice to screen all women and inform them of their immunity status to rubella and offer vaccination to those who are vulnerable to infection.

Since 1970 schoolgirls aged between 11 and 14 have been offered vaccination, but there is considerable variation on the numbers taking advantage of the protection and even those who do cannot be guaranteed permanent immunity. Testing for the presence of antibodies should be undertaken following immunization to ascertain effective results. If the antibody titre is over 1/32 immunity to rubella exists from previous infection. Titres below 1/16 ought to be vaccinated either at the clinic or by the general practitioner. He should be notified in any case so that he is able to inform the clinic of any contraindications before vaccination is given. Attenuated rubella vaccine is injected subcutaneously and pregnancy should be avoided for three months afterwards.

16.5 CONCLUDING COMMENTS

Every person attending a clinic or a general practice for contraception should be aware that pre-pregnancy care is important and available. Knowing that pre-pregnancy care is available encourages the woman to seek advice at a later date when she contemplates embarking on a pregnancy. The majority of prospective parents will probably not require any positive advice but in any case will be reassured to know that they are well prepared. However, a few individuals intelligently guided by health professionals will be able to modify existing hazards and avoid unnecessary disaster. There is therefore little justification for arranging screening programmes larger than the present health care resources can provide. This leaves promotion of desirable standards of pre-pregnancy health to

Table 16.1 The needs of seeds

GOOD STOCK	Genetic inheritance
	Maternal age
	Subfertility
	Miscarriages
POLLINATION	Partner's health
	Partner's fertility
CORRECT SOIL	Normal reproductive organs
AND PLANTING	Menstrual history
	Obstetric history
	Medical history
	Surgical history
	Contraceptive history
FERTILIZER	Body reserves
	Dietary history
	Gastrointestinal illness
PESTS AND	Smoking
ENVIRONMENTAL HAZARDS	Alcohol
	Infection
	Drugs
	Toxic agents
	Pollution
	Poverty

workers in general practice, well-women and family planning clinics, school nurses, health visitors and midwives. Counselling for future pregnancies should form part of all general nursing and medical consultations where disease or its treatment may conflict with the safety of childbearing.

A framework of considerations in pre-pregnancy counselling is given in Table 16.1.

17
Unplanned pregnancy

17.1 DIAGNOSIS OF PREGNANCY

Family planning nurses frequently come across women who think they may be pregnant. There are various reasons for this. A suspected pregnancy is often the deciding factor in motivating a woman to attend a family planning clinic for the first time. Intentions to sort out their contraceptive arrangements are easily deferred by some people until a menstrual irregularity causes them to realize the risks they have been taking in getting involved in an unplanned pregnancy. It should also be remembered that many women using contraceptives are late with their periods, and some have an induced amenorrhoea as a side effect of progestogen therapy. When this occurs they are inclined to jump to the conclusion that they must be pregnant. In all these circumstances it might restore confidence if the nurse can explain to them briefly the signs and symptoms which may be experienced in early pregnancy.

17.2 SYMPTOMS OF PREGNANCY

Pregnancy may be anticipated when a woman who has previously experienced a regular menstrual cycle reports amenorrhoea following unprotected intercourse.

A history of nausea, with or without actual vomiting, at any time during the day is suggestive of pregnancy. Allowances should be made if the woman is highly anxious about a possible pregnancy as the tension and anticipation of an unplanned pregnancy can sometimes cause nausea.

Enlargement and tenderness of the breasts begins quite quickly after the onset of pregnancy and will be noticeable as early as two weeks. The same symptoms may be felt temporarily before periods. The changes in pigmentation of the areola surrounding the nipple in primigravid women are not always present, as fair skinned women rarely develop the darker pigmentation.

Frequency of micturition is a common symptom in early pregnancy and the absence of any discomfort whilst voiding is significant. Care must be taken when enquiring about the frequency of micturition because urethritis and cystitis are very common in sexually active women, and although great discomfort is reported if the infection is acute, some quite low grade infections may cause a degree of frequency without much else in the way of symptoms.

A few women will report changes in appetite and dietary habits and some quite suddenly go off a particular food or beverage and may possibly commence a craving for a particular item such as banana. It is certainly not uncommon to find that coffee has been discontinued as it is found to be nauseating.

Signs of pregnancy are seen and felt later, following the early symptoms. The recognition of fetal movements is usually impossible before 16 weeks and is often as late as 22 weeks especially in a first pregnancy. The enlarged uterus can usually be palpated by 16 weeks and the fetal heart may be heard using an ultrasonic detector as early as 13 weeks although it is necessary for the fundus to be above the symphysis. The fetal heart cannot be heard with an ordinary fetal stethoscope until about 24 weeks when the uterine growth will be level with or above the mother's umbilicus. A pelvic ultrasound scan of the pelvic contents may show a gestation sac in the uterine cavity as early as 2 weeks after the missed period, but this will usually require subsequent investigation to confirm the presence of a fetus.

Simple and quick pregnancy tests can be carried out by testing a specimen of urine for a substance excreted from the cells forming the embryonic sac, beta HCG (human chorionic gonadotrophin). This substance is found in maternal blood and in the urine early in pregnancy and rises quite rapidly reaching a maximum around 16 weeks. Recently, methods of estimating beta HCG in blood have been developed which detect it within a few days of an absent period, but laboratory facilities are necessary. Urine testing for the same beta HCG cannot be contemplated as early, but is considerably simpler. Many clinics have kits for testing urine and this enables women to have a test done at once if her last period was exactly six weeks previously. This immediate action reduces the amount of time which could be wasted in waiting for results if the urine has to be sent for testing to the local hospital pathology department. Because of overnight physiological concentration the first urine to be passed on rising will be most likely to give a positive result and this can be any time after 42 days following the last normal menstrual period. With beta HCG testing kits greater specificity is providing earlier positive results. If the urine is tested too soon, false negative results will be reported and women should be reminded to reattend for further confirmation of their pregnancy status. If a termination is being contemplated then it will be easier and safer if there is the minimum delay in diagnosis and operation. There are many extremely accurate and easy to understand home pregnancy testing kits available for purchase from retail pharmacists, who also provide a pregnancy testing service for those women who would rather not do it themselves.

Examination for pregnancy will be undertaken by the clinic doctor who can examine the woman, and by gentle bimanual examination may find the uterus slightly enlarged and globular in shape and the cervix a softer consistency than usual. Vaginal inspection usually reveals a deeper blue-mauve coloring to the cervix due to the increased vascularity of the pelvic organs occurring early in pregnancy.

17.3 PREGNANCY COUNSELLING

When a pregnancy has been diagnosed it becomes necessary to discuss the results with the woman. It is impossible to anticipate accurately the effect of the news on the woman and immediate reactions vary widely, and may change. It is always a shock to discover that an unplanned pregnancy is already established, and if the woman is single there may be additional problems. The nurse should appreciate that time must be provided to consider the implications of the momentous news. Whatever the woman's feelings at the first impact, allowances must be made for changing feelings. She may ask for arrangements to be made at once for termination, but she is often in no condition to benefit from any counselling at that time. She will, however, appreciate the support and encouragement given to return and discuss what she decides to do.

When she returns to the clinic, a single woman may very well be uncertain and confused about the best possible action. It is helpful if a trained counsellor can arrange to give her time to talk through her feelings. It is also useful for her to have some help in sorting out her feelings, and finding out what actions can be taken, what types of help are available if she wishes to continue with the pregnancy, and receive a realistic outline of the problems facing her in rearing a child alone. The feelings of her partner are also important: he may wish to be involved and, if that is the case, he should not be excluded. Termination need not be discussed in detail until a decision has been made, but if this is the course of action decided upon then an outline of what it may involve will help her to understand what steps are necessary, how and where she can make suitable arrangements for referral and obtain the documents without wasting time, which increases the chances of the pregnancy becoming better established. It is essential that the decision about her pregnancy is made by the woman herself. It is the responsibility of all the personnel involved to see that the woman does not decide to pursue a line of action which has been decided for her by parents, relatives, friends, partner or indeed by her own doctor or the doctors and nurses in the clinic. If there is any ambivalance at any stage in the arrangements for termination, another counselling session should be encouraged and complete freedom given to the woman to entirely reconsider her decision.

A woman who knows her mind on this difficult matter and makes a firm decision recovers well from termination. A few women are very ambivalent from the beginning, and regret the decision. They need support and follow-up attention. If it is not acceptable for the woman to return to the counsellor then she should be referred to her general practitioner.

There are unfortunately a number of women who feel guilty and depressed for many years after the event and who have never found their way to anyone for help. They do, on occasion, unexpectedly display these emotions in the clinic and the nurse should be aware of the possibility of an outbreak of weeping, or recognize a sudden inability to use contraception as a plea for help. The woman, and sometimes her partner also, should be encouraged to attend some sessions with a counsellor skilled in post-abortion depression who may be able to sort out some of the problems. Left untreated it can gradually improve, but in many cases the depression becomes a deep-seated and long-term problem likely to produce serious difficulties.

17.4 TERMINATION OF PREGNANCY

The question of termination may arise at a family planning clinic if a woman finds that the contraceptive technique which she is using has failed. The reasons for failure are numerous and usually difficult to elucidate. In some cases the woman is already pregnant when she first visits the clinic. It is important that advice should be readily available, whether she wishes to continue with the pregnancy or seek a termination, and it is for this reason that the subject is discussed in this section.

In 1967 the Abortion Act formally clarified the legal position of termination of pregnancy in England and Wales. The act became law in Scotland the following year. Since then, if, in the opinion of two registered medical practitioners, a patient qualifies under one or more clauses of the Abortion Act, termination may be performed in a properly licensed hospital or nursing home. (All NHS hospitals with gynaecological operating facilities are automatically licensed places.) Whilst there are obviously moral and ethical aspects of the Act which are open to wide personal interpretation, there are certain legal requirements which must be adhered to before a termination can be performed. An essential document is the green certificate A, which states that two named doctors have seen and examined the woman and are satisfied that termination of pregnancy is justified because it fits into one of the following four groups:

1. The continuance of the pregnancy would involve risk to the life of the pregnant woman greater than if the pregnancy were terminated;
2. The continuance of the pregnancy would involve risk of injury to the physical or mental health of the pregnant woman greater than if the pregnancy were terminated;
3. The continuance of the pregnancy would involve risk of injury to the physical or mental health of the existing child(ren) of the family of the pregnant woman greater than if the pregnancy were terminated;
4. There is substantial risk that if the child were born it would suffer from such physical or mental abnormalities as to be seriously handicapped.

It is mandatory that this certificate is completed and signed before the commencement of treatment for termination of pregnancy to which it refers, and evidence to this extent is given on the form which notifies the operation to the Department of Health (buff coloured certificate HSA 4).

Abortion falls into two main operative groups depending on the gestational age of the pregnancy: up to 12 weeks' and over 12 weeks' gestation. At present the latter group extends right up to 28 weeks, the date of legal viability. Complications have occurred lately because it is now quite possible to keep premature infants of 26 weeks alive, and the assessment of legal viability must be set to an earlier gestation because of advances in neonatal medical achievements. Much parliamentary discussion has been aimed at reducing the upper limit for termination to 18 weeks, but this would severely limit therapeutic abortion following amniocentesis for fetal abnormality where the results may not be available until a later date. The report of the working committee on the Abortion Act 1974 suggested an upper limit of 24 weeks, and this would seem to represent the limit between ability of the fetus to survive independently of the mother and leave time for the results of tests for fetal abnormality to be available. Only in exceptional circumstances related to abnormality is termination justified after 18 weeks but clinical freedom should be allowed for the fetus with chromosomal abnormalities which take time to diagnose.

Facilities available for termination

Any woman wishing to arrange termination of pregnancy should be advised to see her own family doctor and if he agrees to accede to her request it will be necessary for him to refer her to another doctor, usually a gynaecologist, for a second opinion. Very occasionally, personal moral considerations may prevent advice being given and in this situation the doctor usually refers the woman to another doctor who is prepared to undertake her case. Similarly, nurses may also find that their own views are too strong to allow them to give impartial advice, and if this is the case they too should arrange for a nurse colleague to deal with the case.

The operation of termination of pregnancy can only be undertaken in those places licensed by the Department of Health. Facilities exist in most NHS hospitals and a small number of private clinics, some of which are run by recognized charities, whilst others are entirely independent. Conditions vary considerably throughout the country. There may well be some geographical limitations of termination availability inside the National Health Service. Even where facilities exist, the operation may not be performed because of religious or moral attitudes, but the service throughout the United Kingdom is gradually becoming more evenly distributed. Still, in a hard-pressed NHS there is a limit on the number of termination operations which can be fitted in without disrupting the standards of other gynaecological care, and advice may need to be given to women about approaching a sound charitable organization. These organizations are usually non-profitmaking and some run their own counselling service, nursing homes and operating theatres. There is a fixed charge which covers all fees for medical examination, blood tests, operation and nursing home services, and on the whole the standards set are high. Indeed, they are run very efficiently and have the extra advantage for the patient of receiving care without the distress of meeting terminally ill and infertile patients who could share a hospital ward. The family doctor may refer the patient to one of these organizations or a termination may be privately arranged.

Methods of termination

In early pregnancy the contents of the uterus can be aspirated under general anaesthetic. Later terminations, after 13 weeks, may be managed by inducing uterine contractions with prostaglandin substances. Only very occasionally nowadays would an hysterotomy, an abdominal operation which removes the fetus, prove to be necessary.

Aspiration termination
The method of termination by dilating the cervix and using a suction catheter to evacuate the uterine contents is effective up to 13 weeks' gestation. It is usually performed under a general anaesthetic, or more rarely in the earliest pregnancies using a paracervical nerve block.

At operation the uterus is assessed so that the correct size of aspirating cannula can be chosen. Disposable plastic Karman cannulae are available in various sizes up to 12 gauge and the size 10 is usually suitable for evacuating up to a 12 week gestation. Metal Biera cannulae are also available and the larger sizes are suitable for later termination.

Graded dilators are passed through the cervix so that the

opening is gradually enlarged to be just slightly bigger than the suction cannula which has been chosen. It has been shown that whilst termination can be performed at stages later than 13 weeks by the vaginal approach, the amount of dilation required is likely to cause permanent damage to the circular muscle ring known as the internal cervical os, and this can result in mid-trimester abortion or premature labour in subsequent pregnancies.

The suction cannulae are attached to a high power vacuum and are moved up and down to cover the entire lining of the uterus so that the contents are completely aspirated. Final confirmation that the uterine cavity is empty is achieved by careful sharp currettage, when no further bleeding should occur. Post-operatively the blood loss should not necessitate the use of more than three or four sanitary towels during the first eight hours, and normal menstrual protection thereafter for perhaps a day or two. If the bleeding is heavier then 0.5 mg ergometrine may be given by intramuscular injection. Some supra-pubic abdominal pain is usual for one or two hours following the operation and is rather more likely in those women who usually suffer from dysmennorhoea; it rarely causes distress. Analgesia should, however, be available if and when necessary. Occasionally the uterine fundus is palpable and this suggests that it may have become distended with a blood clot which should be spontaneously expelled.

Possible complications include excessive bleeding, perforation of the uterus and later sepsis. It is not unusual for prophylactic antibiotics to be given to prevent the possibility of intrauterine infection developing and causing chronic complications.

Later termination

No matter how much publicity is given to encourage women to seek advice early, there is always a small proportion whose request for termination comes later than 13 weeks' gestation. Delay is sometimes due to a slow system of referral and if this is the case the system needs to be reappraised. Some women request termination when screening tests carried out in pregnancy prove fetal abnormality or death. Unfortunately these tests take time to confirm and these inevitable delays cause a later termination to become necessary. The recent introduction of chorion villus biopsy as an alternative to amniocentesis in the detection of chromosomal and biochemical abnormalities will help to reduce the number of later terminations but there will still be a requirement. Another group of late referrals are teenagers who have kept the accident to themselves for fear of discussion with parents or who have genuinely been unaware of the reason for the absence of their periods. They create a special problem and are discussed in the chapter on special needs.

Later terminations may be managed by prostaglandin which induces uterine contractions and expulsion of the fetus like a spontaneous miscarriage. This is now the method of choice. There are many varieties of this hormone found in all body cells. Preparations of prostaglandin, now made synthetically, are effective in causing uterine action even early in pregnancy although there may be some delay after administration before it begins to take effect.

Prostaglandin is given either as a gel when it is inserted through the cervix using a soft catheter, or it may be injected directly into the amniotic sac through the abdominal and uterine walls under local anaesthetic. Contractions will commence, but sometimes not for several hours, and the fetus is eventually delivered vaginally in a similar way to miscarriage or premature delivery. The placenta is frequently retained owing to its failure to separate from the uterine anchorage. Analgesia is necessary in most cases because the uterine contractions are distressing and may continue for 8–24 hours. An epidural anaesthetic, when this is available, will give the best relief from pain. Some form of analgesia, moral support and privacy should always be provided.

Complications of prostaglandin termination may include nausea, vomiting and diarrhoea as in its present forms prostaglandin is irritating to the whole gastro-intestinal tract. Intrauterine infection may follow any termination as can haemorrhage. Unfortunately it is common for placental tissue to be retained after the expulsion of the fetus and a D and C is usually necessary and requires a general anaesthetic. Uterine rupture and cervical laceration may occur if the contractions are very strong, but fortunately these are rare complications.

Just occasionally the woman does not respond to prostaglandins, even when reinforced with syntocinon, and the uterus will not contract; and this may necessitate hysterotomy. Luckily with modern techniques this operation is almost a thing of the past. It involves removing the fetus through an incision in the uterus, but this leaves a scar on the uterus which will form a weakness in subsequent pregnancies and a scarred reminder on the abdominal wall. The requirement for this procedure is fortunately rare and the decision to operate would almost certainly rest with a consultant gynaecologist.

A few women will need support following their termination and discharge from hospital and they should be advised to contact their family doctor who will either offer support himself or ask a health visitor to do so. Help is provided by most health visitors if they are made aware of the need to visit.

18

Future developments

18.1 THE MALE PILL

Before this method can become established there are social as well as biological hurdles. Will the man comply with the regime and will his partner be able to trust what he tells her as the implications of failure only affect her body?

It is possible to suppress sperm formation using androgens and progestogens, and the most promising combination is a monthly injection of 200 mg depo-medroxyprogesterone and 250 mg testosterone enanthate, which is undergoing a WHO multi-centre trial. Problems with this method centre on the immense number of sperm and continuous chain of production. The sperm reservoir has to be emptied by ejaculation over a considerable time in exactly the same way as post-vasectomy.

A less attractive alternative is Gossypol, which was identified in cotton seed oil when scientists were investigating an epidemic of male subfertility in China. This substance inhibits sperm formation and eventually stops production completely but the effect is not yet guaranteed as reversible, and has highly toxic side effects.

Work has been undertaken on an anti-FSH substance which inhibits both spermatogenesis and ovulation, and this raises the prospect of a 'his or her's' pill.

Spermicides

The motility of sperm can be reduced so that they are unable to penetrate the cervical mucus by placing a gel containing the well-known antihypertensive propranolol in the woman's vagina. Whilst this method appears promising it depends on action being

taken by the woman rather than the man and cannot be truly described as male contraception.

18.2 FEMALE CONTRACEPTION

Systemic methods

There have been several new progestogens recently developed, for
instance Gestodene which has no androgenic activity and causes
minimal metabolic disturbance. It has recently been marketed as a
combined oral contraceptive under the name of Femodene. Further
attention is being paid to norgestimate which has a strong
antiovulatory effect because of its anti-FSH action. It seems to
provide good cycle control and is already available on the
continent.

It is possible to obtain preparations with an antiprogestogenic
effect, and mifepristone seems to be the most likely to become
commercially available. These substances can disrupt both ovulation and the luteal phase of the cycle, and could be used for
interruption of early pregnancies before five weeks gestation.

Peptide contraception could be a safe and effective alternative
to steroid contraception. Over-stimulation of the pituitary by
administering an excess of LH releasing hormone peptides results
in a refractory period when production of FSH and LH ceases.
This can either be used on a cyclical basis, as an implant or post-
coitally. The method is unlikely to be available in the near future
and is likely to be quite expensive.

New hormone delivery systems

Whilst the progestasert IUD was short-lived, research has continued along these lines and with the availability of levonorgestrel
a new attempt has been made to construct a device similar to the
Novagard, but with a wider stem which releases 20 mg per day. As
efficacy lasts for approximately five years the drawback of the
progestasert needing replacement every twelve months has been
overcome.

Vaginal rings made of a hollow silastic material filled with
progestogen can be inserted in the vagina and are effective for up
to 90 days. The fitting does not need to be particularly accurate
although there is obviously a best size for retention and comfort.

The ring remains in situ during intercourse and whilst menstruating and the advantage lies in the released hormone being absorbed locally and not needing to pass through the hepatic circulation, and there is no likelihood of gastrointestinal disorders disrupting the effectiveness. If this method becomes more widely used and acceptable then developments concerned with implants beneath the skin will be unlikely to continue because of the disadvantages of minor surgery.

A female condom

Research into a female condom is complete and this should be available commercially in a short while. The condom consists of a polyurethane bag with two rings: the upper acting like a diaphragm ring whilst the lower ring covers the vulva and prevents the condom riding upwards during intercourse. The advantage of protection from sexually transmitted diseases should make the method popular and unlike the diaphragm it does not need accurate placing to be certain of complete occlusion of the cervix.

18.3 CONCLUSION

Fears are frequently raised about the ever-increasing world population: more infants survive to adulthood and death is occurring later. To avoid stretching resources, the cry for family planning is raised but, however helpful any national programme may be with regard to finance, in influencing opinion it is the health worker taking the information to an individual or family who carries the torch. Demography is the concern of governments: family planning the concern of informed individuals. In this text the aim has been to prepare health professionals to convey accurate and helpful information. The quality of personal life must benefit from people's ability to limit their own progeny without limiting their natural instincts, and thus contribute intelligently to the wider call for co-existence with all other forms of life.

Further reading

GENERAL

Christopher, E. (1988) *Sexuality and Birth Control in Social and Community Work*. Temple Smith, London.

Delvin, D. (1979) *The Book of Love*. New English Library, London.

Ford, A. (1985) *Men*. Corgi, London.

Llewlyn-Jones, D. (1980) *Everywoman*. Faber, London.

Llewlyn-Jones, D. (1987) *Everyman*. Oxford University Press, Oxford.

Louden, N. (1985) *The Handbook of Family Planning*. Churchill Livingstone, Edinburgh.

Zilbergeld, B. (1984) *Men and Sex*. Fontana Collins, London.

COUNSELLING AND SEXUALITY

Balint, M. (1980) *The Doctor, the Patient and his Illness*. Pitman, London.

Bancroft, J. (1983) *Human Sexuality and its Problems*. Churchill Livingstone, Edinburgh.

Savage, J. (1987) *Nurses, Gender and Sexuality*. Heinemann Nursing, London.

Tschudin, V. (1982) *Counselling Skills for Nurses*. Balliere Tindall, London.

Tunnadine, D. (1978) *Unplanned Pregnancy, Accident or Illness?* Oxford University Press, Oxford.

Tunnadine, L.P.D. (1985) *The Making of Love*. Unwin, London.

Webb, C. (1985) *Sexuality, Nursing and Health*. John Wiley and Sons, Chichester.

LEGAL

Paxman, J. (1980) *The Law and Planned Parenthood*. IPPF, London.

HISTORY

Evans, B. (1987) *Freedom to Choose*. Bodley Head, London.

Leathard, A. (1980) *The Fight for Family Planning*. Macmillan, London.

McLaren, A. (1978) *Birth Control in Nineteenth Century England*. Croom Helm, London.

Wood, C. and Sutters, B. (1970) *Fight for Acceptance, a History of Contraception*. MTP Press, Lancaster.

METHODS OF CONTRACEPTION

Flynn, A. and Brooks, M. (1984) *The Manual of Natural Family Planning*. George Allen Unwin, Boston.

Goldstein, M. and Feldberg, M. (1985) *The Vasectomy Book*. Tunstone Press, Wellingborough.

Guillebaud, J. (1984) *The Pill*. Oxford University Press, Oxford.

FERTILITY AND SUBFERTILITY

Borg, S. and Lasker, J. (1982) *When Pregnancy Fails*. Routledge and Kegan Paul, London.

Hull, M. (1981) *Clinics in Obstetrics and Gynaecology*. Vol. 8, No. 3. W.B. Saunders, Eastbourne.

Llewlyn-Jones, D. (1985) *Fundamentals of Gynaecology*. Faber, London.

Pizer, H. and Palinski, C. (1980) *Coping with Miscarriage*. Jill Norman, London.

WELL WOMEN

Sandford, C. (1983) *Enjoy Sex in the Middle Years*. Marriage Guidance Council, London.

INFECTION

Oakes, J. (1983) *Herpes, The Facts*. Penguin, Harmondsworth.

Llewlyn-Jones, D. *Herpes and Other Sexually Transmitted Diseases*. Faber, London.

PRECONCEPTUAL CARE

Chamberlain, G. and Lumley, J. (1986) *Prepregnancy Care*. John Wiley and Sons, Chichester.

Hailey, J. (1982) *Clinics in Obstetrics and Gynaecology*. Vol. 9, No. 1. W.B. Saunders, Eastbourne.

SPECIAL NEEDS

Close, S. (1984) *Sex During Pregnancy and After Childbirth*. Thorsons, Wellingborough.

Gill, D. (1977) *Illegitimacy, Sexuality and the Status of Women*. Blackwell, Oxford.

Hart, J. and Richardson, D. (1984) *Theory and Practice of Homosexuality*. Routledge and Kegan Paul, London.

Henley, A. (1979) *Asian Patients in Hospital and At Home*. King's Fund, London.

Mooney, T., Cole, T. and Chilgrin, R. (1975) *Sexual Options for Paraplegics*. Little, Brown and Co., Boston, MA.

Stewart, W. (1979) *The Sexual Side of Handicap*. Woodhead-Faulkener, Cambridge.

Task Force on Concerns of the Physically Handicapped (1978) *Towards Intimacy*. Human Sciences Press, New York; European Distributors Eurospan Ltd, London.

Index